ORTHOPEDIC CLINICS OF NORTH AMERICA

www.orthopedic.theclinics.com

Orthopedic Urgencies and Emergencies

July 2016 • Volume 47 • Number 3

Editors

JAMES H. CALANDRUCCIO
BENJAMIN J. GREAR
BENJAMIN M. MAUCK
JEFFREY R. SAWYER
PATRICK C. TOY
JOHN C. WEINLEIN

ELSEVIER

1600 John F. Kennedy Boulevard • Suite 1800 • Philadelphia, Pennsylvania, 19103-2899.

http://www.orthopedic.theclinics.com

ORTHOPEDIC CLINICS OF NORTH AMERICA Volume 47, Number 3
July 2016 ISSN 0030-5898, ISBN-13: 978-0-323-44850-5

Editor: Jennifer Flynn-Briggs
Developmental Editor: Kristen Helm

Orthopedic Clinics of North America (ISSN 0030-5898) is published quarterly by Elsevier Inc., 360 Park Avenue South, New York, NY 10010-1710. Months of issue are January, April, July, and October. Business and Editorial Offices: 1600 John F. Kennedy Blvd., Suite 1800, Philadelphia, PA 19103-2899. Customer Service Office: 3251 Riverport Lane, Maryland Heights, MO 63043. Periodicals postage paid at New York, NY and additional mailing offices. Subscription prices are $310.00 per year for (US individuals), $653.00 per year for (US institutions), $365.00 per year (Canadian individuals), $797.00 per year (Canadian institutions), $450.00 per year (international individuals), $797.00 per year (international institutions), $100.00 per year (US students), $220.00 per year (Canadian and international students). Foreign air speed delivery is included in all *Clinics* subscription prices. All prices are subject to change without notice. **POSTMASTER: Send change of address to** *Orthopedic Clinics of North America,* **Elsevier Health Sciences Division, Subscription Customer Service, 3251 Riverport Lane, Maryland Heights, MO 63043. Customer Service (orders, claims, online, change of address): Elsevier Health Sciences Division, Subscription Customer Service, 3251 Riverport Lane, Maryland Heights, MO 63043. Tel: 1-800-654-2452 (U.S. and Canada); 314-447-8871 (outside U.S. and Canada). Fax: 314-447-8029. E-mail:** journalscustomerservice-usa@elsevier.com **(for print support);** journalsonlinesupport-usa@elsevier.com **(for online support).**

Reprints. For copies of 100 or more, of articles in this publication, please contact the Commercial Reprints Department, Elsevier Inc., 360 Park Avenue South, New York, NY 10010-1710. Tel.: 212-633-3874; Fax: 212-633-3820; E-mail: reprints@elsevier.com.

Orthopedic Clinics of North America is covered in *MEDLINE/PubMed* (*Index Medicus*), *Cinahl, Excerpta Medica, and Cumulative Index to Nursing and Allied Health Literature.*

PROGRAM OBJECTIVE

Orthopedic Clinics of North America offers clinical review articles on the most cutting-edge technologies and techniques in the field, including adult reconstruction, the upper extremity, pediatrics, trauma, oncology, and sports medicine.

TARGET AUDIENCE

Practicing orthopedic surgeons, orthopedic residents, and other healthcare professionals who specialize in orthopedic technologies and techniques for adult reconstruction, the upper extremity, pediatrics, trauma, oncology, and sports medicine.

LEARNING OBJECTIVES

Upon completion of this activity, participants will be able to:
1. Review the emergency treatment of compartment syndrome in children and adults.
2. Discuss the evaluation of emergent pediatric conditions, including open fractures.
3. Recognize the diagnosis and management of urgent and emergent orthopedic conditions of the upper and lower extremity.

ACCREDITATION

The Elsevier Office of Continuing Medical Education (EOCME) is accredited by the Accreditation Council for Continuing Medical Education (ACCME) to provide continuing medical education for physicians.

The EOCME designates this enduring material for a maximum of 15 *AMA PRA Category 1 Credit*(s)™. Physicians should claim only the credit commensurate with the extent of their participation in the activity.

All other health care professionals requesting continuing education credit for this enduring material will be issued a certificate of participation.

DISCLOSURE OF CONFLICTS OF INTEREST

The EOCME assesses conflict of interest with its instructors, faculty, planners, and other individuals who are in a position to control the content of CME activities. All relevant conflicts of interest that are identified are thoroughly vetted by EOCME for fair balance, scientific objectivity, and patient care recommendations. EOCME is committed to providing its learners with CME activities that promote improvements or quality in healthcare and not a specific proprietary business or a commercial interest.

The planning committee, staff, authors and editors listed below have identified no financial relationships or relationships to products or devices they or their spouse/life partner have with commercial interest related to the content of this CME activity:

Reid A. Abrams, MD; Jennifer M. Bauer, MD; Michael J. Beebe, MD; Tyler A. Cannon, MD; Priscilla K. Cavanaugh, MD; Mohammad A. Enayatollahi, MD; Safa Cyrus Fassihi, BS; Jennifer Flynn-Briggs; Anjali Fortna; Jonathan D. Gillig, MD; Benjamin J. Grear, MD; Christopher B. Hayes, MD; Martin J. Herman, MD; Pooya Hosseinzadeh, MD; Mitchell G. Maltenfort, PhD, MBA; Hassan R. Mir, MD, MBA, FACS; Premkumar Nandhakumar; Nikhil R. Oak, MD; Javad Parvizi, MD, FRCS; James Nicholas Rachel, MD; Camilo Restrepo, MD; Megan Suermann; Kostas M. Triantafillou, MD; Arianna Trionfo, MD; Derek Ward, MD; Stephen D. White, MD.

The planning committee, staff, authors and editors listed below have identified financial relationships or relationships to products or devices they or their spouse/life partner have with commercial interest related to the content of this CME activity:

William C. Pederson, MD, FACS receives royalties/patents from Elsevier B.V.
Matthew I. Rudloff, MD is on the speakers' bureau for Smith & Nephew, and receives royalties/patents from Elsevier B.V.
Andrew H. Schmidt, MD is a consultant/advisor for Acumed, A Colson Associate; and Conventus Orthopaedics, has stock ownership in EPIX Orthopedics, Inc.; EPIEN Medical, Inc.; and Twin Star Medical, and receives royalties from Thieme Medical Publishers, Inc. His spouse/partner is a consultant/advisor for St. Jude Medical, Inc.

UNAPPROVED/OFF-LABEL USE DISCLOSURE

The EOCME requires CME faculty to disclose to the participants:
1. When products or procedures being discussed are off-label, unlabelled, experimental, and/or investigational (not US Food and Drug Administration [FDA] approved); and
2. Any limitations on the information presented, such as data that are preliminary or that represent ongoing research, interim analyses, and/or unsupported opinions. Faculty may discuss information about pharmaceutical agents that is outside of FDA-approved labelling. This information is intended solely for CME and is not intended to promote off-label use of these medications. If you have any questions, contact the medical affairs department of the manufacturer for the most recent prescribing information.

TO ENROLL

To enroll in the *Orthopedic Clinics of North America* Continuing Medical Education program, call customer service at 1-800-654-2452 or sign up online at http://www.theclinics.com/home/cme. The CME program is available to subscribers for an additional annual fee of USD 215.

METHOD OF PARTICIPATION

In order to claim credit, participants must complete the following:
1. Complete enrolment as indicated above.
2. Read the activity.
3. Complete the CME Test and Evaluation. Participants must achieve a score of 70% on the test. All CME Tests and Evaluations must be completed online.

CME INQUIRIES/SPECIAL NEEDS

For all CME inquiries or special needs, please contact elsevierCME@elsevier.com.

EDITORIAL BOARD

CONTRIBUTORS

AUTHORS

REID A. ABRAMS, MD
Chief, Hand, Upper Extremity, and
Microvascular Surgery; Professor and Vice
Chair, Department of Orthopaedic Surgery,
University of California, San Diego, San Diego,
California

JENNIFER M. BAUER, MD
Orthopaedic Surgery and Rehabilitation,
Vanderbilt University, Nashville, Tennessee

MICHAEL J. BEEBE, MD
Orthopaedic Trauma Service, Florida
Orthopaedic Institute, Tampa, Florida

TYLER A. CANNON, MD
Orthopaedic Surgeon, Tabor Orthopedics and
Faculty at University of Tennessee Health
Science Center, Memphis, Tennessee

PRISCILLA K. CAVANAUGH, MD
Department of Orthopaedic Surgery,
St Christopher's Hospital for Children, Drexel
University College of Medicine, Philadelphia,
Pennsylvania

MOHAMMAD A. ENAYATOLLAHI, MD
Rothman Institute, Thomas Jefferson
University Hospital, Philadelphia,
Pennsylvania

SAFA CYRUS FASSIHI, BS
Rothman Institute, Thomas Jefferson
University Hospital, Philadelphia,
Pennsylvania

JONATHAN D. GILLIG, MD
Department of Orthopaedic Surgery,
University of South Alabama School of
Medicine, Mobile, Alabama

BENJAMIN J. GREAR, MD
Clinical Instructor, Department of
Orthopaedic Surgery and Biomedical
Engineering, University of Tennessee-
Campbell Clinic, Memphis, Tennessee

CHRISTOPHER B. HAYES, MD
Resident Physician, Department of
Orthopedics, University of Kentucky,
Lexington, Kentucky

MARTIN J. HERMAN, MD
Department of Orthopaedic Surgery,
St Christopher's Hospital for Children, Drexel
University College of Medicine, Philadelphia,
Pennsylvania

POOYA HOSSEINZADEH, MD
Assistant Professor, Department of
Orthopedics, Herbert Wertheim College of
Medicine, Baptist Children's Hospital, Florida
International University, Miami, Florida

MITCHELL G. MALTENFORT, PhD, MBA
Rothman Institute, Thomas Jefferson
University Hospital, Philadelphia,
Pennsylvania

HASSAN R. MIR, MD, MBA, FACS
Orthopaedic Trauma Service, Florida
Orthopaedic Institute, Tampa, Florida

NIKHIL R. OAK, MD
Hand, Upper Extremity, and Microvascular
Surgery Fellow, Department of Orthopaedic
Surgery, University of California, San Diego,
San Diego, California

JAVAD PARVIZI, MD, FRCS
James Edwards Professor of Orthopedic
Surgery, Sidney Kimmel Medical College;
Director of Clinical Research, Rothman
Institute, Thomas Jefferson University
Hospital, Philadelphia, Pennsylvania

WILLIAM C. PEDERSON, MD, FACS
Professor of Surgery, Orthopaedics, and
Pediatrics, Baylor College of Medicine;
Head of Hand Surgery and Microsurgery,
Texas Children's Hospital, Houston, Texas

JAMES NICHOLAS RACHEL, MD
Associate Professor, Department of
Orthopaedic Surgery, University of South
Alabama School of Medicine; Elbow, Hand
and Wrist Specialist, The Orthopaedic Group,
PC, Mobile, Alabama

CAMILO RESTREPO, MD
Rothman Institute, Thomas Jefferson
University Hospital, Philadelphia, Pennsylvania

MATTHEW I. RUDLOFF, MD
Assistant Professor, Department of
Orthopaedic Surgery, University of
Tennessee-Campbell Clinic, Memphis,
Tennessee

ANDREW H. SCHMIDT, MD
Chief, Department of Orthopaedic Surgery,
Hennepin County Medical Center; Professor,
Department of Orthopaedic Surgery,
University of Minnesota, Minneapolis,
Minnesota

KOSTAS M. TRIANTAFILLOU, MD
University Orthopedic Surgeons,
University of Tennessee Medical Center,
Knoxville, Tennessee

ARIANNA TRIONFO, MD
Department of Orthopaedic Surgery,
Temple University School of Medicine,
Philadelphia, Pennsylvania

DEREK WARD, MD
Fellow, Adult Reconstruction,
Rothman Institute, Thomas Jefferson
University Hospital, Philadelphia,
Pennsylvania

STEPHEN D. WHITE, MD
Department of Orthopaedic Surgery,
University of South Alabama School of
Medicine, Mobile, Alabama

CONTENTS

Adult Reconstruction
Patrick C. Toy

The diagnosis and treatment of hip pain in the young adult remain a challenge. Recently, understanding of a few specific hip conditions has improved, most notably femoroacetabular impingement. The differential diagnosis of hip pain has also expanded significantly, offering new challenges and opportunities. Along with the diagnostic dilemma, optimal treatment strategies for many conditions have yet to be proven and are current areas of important inquiry. This article reviews the current research on hip pain in the young adult and presents an overview of diagnostic and management strategies.

Studies suggest that total hip arthroplasty (THA) performed through direct anterior (DA) approach has better functional outcomes than other surgical approaches. The immediate to very early outcomes of DA THA are not known. A prospective, randomized study examined the very early outcome of THA performed through DA versus direct lateral approach. The functional outcomes on day 1, day 2, week 6, week 12, 6 months, and 1 year were measured. Patients receiving DA THA had significantly higher functional scores during the early period following surgery. The difference in functional scores leveled out at 6 months.

The diagnosis of periprosthetic joint infection (PJI) following total hip arthroplasty and total knee arthroplasty has been one of the major challenges in orthopedic surgery. As there is no single absolute test for diagnosis of PJI, diagnostic criteria for PJI have been proposed that include using several diagnostic modalities. Focused history, physical examination, plain radiographs, and initial serologic tests should be followed by joint aspiration and synovial analysis. Newer diagnostic techniques, such as alpha-defensin and interleukin-6, hold great promise in the future diagnosis of equivocal infections.

Trauma
John C. Weinlein

Acute compartment syndrome (ACS) is a well-known pathophysiologic complication of trauma or tissue ischemia. ACS affects the appearance, function, and even the viability of the involved limb, and demands immediate diagnosis and treatment. However, ACS is difficult to diagnose and the only effective treatment is decompressive surgical fasciotomy. The clinical signs and symptoms may easily be attributed to other aspects of the injury, which further complicates the diagnosis. This article highlights the latest information regarding the diagnosis of ACS, how to perform fasciotomies, and how to manage fasciotomy wounds, and also reviews complications and outcomes of ACS.

Hip dislocations, most often caused by motor vehicle accidents or similar high-energy trauma, comprise a large subset of distinct injury patterns. Understanding these patterns and their associated injuries allows surgeons to provide optimal care for these patients both in the early and late postinjury periods. Nonoperative care requires surgeons to understand the indications. Surgical care requires the surgeon to understand the benefits and limitations of several surgical approaches. This article presents the current understanding of hip dislocation treatment, focusing on anatomy, injury classifications, nonoperative and operative management, and postinjury care.

High-energy pelvic ring injuries can represent life-threatening injuries in the polytraumatized patient, particularly when presenting with hemodynamic instability. These injuries mandate a systematic multidisciplinary approach to evaluation and timely intervention to address hemorrhage while concomitantly addressing mechanical instability. These pelvic injuries are associated with potentially lethal hemorrhage originating from venous, arterial, and osseous sources. A thorough understanding of anatomy, radiographic findings, and initial physical examination can alert one to the presence of pelvic instability necessitating emergent treatment. The focus is on hemorrhage control, using techniques for skeletal stabilization, angiography, and open procedures to decrease mortality in this high-risk patient population.

Pediatrics
Jeffrey R. Sawyer

Open fractures in children are rare and are typically associated with better prognoses compared with their adult equivalents. Regardless, open fractures pose a challenge because of the risk of healing complications and infection, leading to significant morbidity even in the pediatric population. Therefore, the management of pediatric open fractures requires special consideration.

This article comprehensively reviews the initial evaluation, classification, treatment, outcomes, and controversies of open fractures in children.

Compartment syndrome in children can present differently than in adults. Increased analgesic need should be considered the first sign of evolving compartment syndrome in children. Children with supracondylar humeral fractures, floating elbow injuries, operatively treated forearm fractures, and tibial fractures are at high risk for developing compartment syndrome. Elbow flexion beyond 90° in supracondylar humeral fractures and closed treatment of forearm fractures in floating elbow injuries are associated with increased risk of compartment syndrome. Prompt diagnosis and treatment with fasciotomy in children result in excellent long-term outcomes.

Upper Extremity
Benjamin M. Mauck and James H. Calandruccio

Ischemia of the upper extremity is uncommon but can occur with open or closed trauma. Those dealing with traumatic injury of the upper extremity should be conversant with techniques of vascular surgery and microsurgery to address these injuries when they occur. Closed injury can occur as well, and at times these are best managed nonoperatively. This article discusses the management of both in the acute setting.

Acute carpal tunnel syndrome is a progressive median nerve compression leading to loss of two-point discrimination. Most cases are encountered in the emergency department following wrist trauma and distal radial fractures. Although rare, atraumatic etiologies have been reported, and diligent evaluation of these patients should be performed. If missed or neglected, irreversible damage to the median nerve may result. Once diagnosed, emergent carpal tunnel release should be performed. If performed in a timely manner, outcomes are excellent, often with complete recovery.

Hand compartment syndrome has many etiologies; untreated, it has dire functional consequences. Intracompartmental pressure exceeding capillary filling pressure causes decreased tissue perfusion resulting in progressive ischemic death of compartment contents. Clinical findings can evolve. Serial physical examinations are recommended and, if equivocal, interstitial pressure monitoring is indicated. Definitive management is emergent fasciotomies with incisions designed to decompress the involved hand compartments, which could include the thenar, hypothenar, and interosseous compartments, and the carpal tunnel. Careful wound care, edema management, splinting, and hand therapy are critical. Therapy should start early postoperatively, possibly before wound closure.

High-pressure injection hand injuries are often overlooked, with severe complications owing to the acute inflammatory response. Prognosis depends on the type of material injected, location of injection, involved pressure, and timing to surgical decompression and debridement. Acute management involves broad-spectrum antibiotics, tetanus prophylaxis, emergent decompression within 6 hours, and complete removal of the injected material. Most patients have residual sequelae of stiffness, pain, sensation loss, and difficulties in returning to work. The hand surgeon's role is prompt surgical intervention, early postoperative motion, and education of patient and staff regarding short- and long-term expectations.

Foot and Ankle
Benjamin J. Grear

This review article provides an overview of talus fractures. Special attention is given to the clinical literature that evaluates the timing of surgical management for displaced talus fractures. Several series support delayed definitive fixation for talus fractures, suggesting displaced fractures do not necessitate emergent surgical fixation.

ORTHOPEDIC URGENCIES AND EMERGENCIES

THE CLINICS ARE AVAILABLE ONLINE!

Access your subscription at:
www.theclinics.com

Erratum

In the January 2015 issue of *Orthopedic Clinics* (Volume 46, Issue 1), in the article "Patellar Instability" by Jason L. Koh and Cory Stewart, an error was made regarding the various patella height ratios. Figure 1 explains methods of measuring the patellar height ratios, wherein all three methods (Insall-Salvati, Caton-Deschamps, Blackburne-Peel) are mentioned as ratios between the articular surface of the patella and its distance with tibia, i.e., patella:tendon. In the original descriptions by the aforementioned authors, the ratios are calculated as indices of tendon:patella.

The authors apologize for this error.

Orthop Clin N Am 47 (2016) xv
http://dx.doi.org/10.1016/j.ocl.2016.04.002
0030-5898/16/$ – see front matter © 2016 Elsevier Inc. All rights reserved.

ERRATUM

PREFACE

Orthopedic Urgencies and Emergencies

Ever wonder where the line between urgency and emergency falls? Sometimes, it's difficult to tell. Orthopedic injuries are commonly seen in both emergent and urgent care settings. Common presentations can mimic serious conditions.

The authors of these sections have provided much useful information on this topic that can help surgeons deal with these urgencies and emergencies. All of these articles contain much information from experienced surgeons in orthopedics, and we thank them for providing their wisdom.

Articles in the Adult Reconstruction Section will focus on the following: Management of Hip Pain in Young Adults, Total Hip Arthroplasty Performed through Direct Anterior Approach Provides Superior Early Outcome, and Diagnosis of Periprosthetic Joint Infection Following Hip and Knee Arthroplasty.

Articles in the Trauma Section will focus on the following: Acute Compartment Syndrome, Treatment of Hip Dislocations and Associated Injuries,

and Management of Pelvic Ring Injuries in Unstable Patients.

Articles in the Pediatrics Section will focus on the following: Pediatric Open Fractures, and Compartment Syndrome in Children.

Articles in the Upper Extremity Section will focus on the following: Acute Ischemia of the Upper Extremity, Acute Carpal Tunnel Syndrome, Compartment Syndrome of the Hand, and High-Pressure Injection Injuries of the Hand.

Articles in the Foot and Ankle Section will focus on the following: Review of Talus Fractures and Surgical Timing.

I hope that our readers will find this material useful.

Jennifer Flynn-Briggs
Senior Clinics Editor, Elsevier

E-mail address:
j.flynn-briggs@elsevier.com

Orthop Clin N Am 47 (2016) xvii
http://dx.doi.org/10.1016/j.ocl.2016.04.001
0030-5898/16/$ – see front matter © 2016 Published by Elsevier Inc.

Adult Reconstruction

Management of Hip Pain in Young Adults

Derek Ward, MD, Javad Parvizi, MD, FRCS*

Derek Ward, MD, Javad Parvizi, MD, FRCS*

KEYWORDS

• Hip pain • Femoroacetabular impingement • Dysplasia

KEY POINTS

• Differential diagnosis of hip and groin pain.
• Nonoperative treatments of hip pain.
• Operative treatments of hip pain.
• Current concepts in management of femoroacetabular impingement.

INTRODUCTION

The management of hip pain in the young adult remains a challenge in some circumstances. Over the past few decades, understanding of a few specific conditions affecting the hip has advanced. Femoroacetabular impingement (FAI) is a condition that was popularized in recent decades. The optimal management of FAI and many other conditions affecting the hip is still unknown. The differential diagnosis of hip pain has also expanded, bringing with it new challenges and opportunities. The management of various causes affecting the labrum and cartilage of the hip joint are particularly problematic in the young patient, and evolution of the understanding of the young adult hip has dramatically changed management of this patient population. This article reviews the current literature on hip pain in young adults (ages 18–35 years), including physical and imaging diagnosis, the accepted treatments and controversies, and areas for further progress.

EVALUATION OF HIP PAIN IN THE YOUNG ADULT

Clinical Presentation

A careful history and physical examination should be performed to appropriately elucidate the cause of the patient's symptoms. The location of the pain is important because intra-articular hip pain most commonly presents in the groin but may also present on the side of the hip, in the buttock, and may refer to the anteromedial knee via the obturator nerve. Patients with FAI or other intra-articular pathologic condition may make a c-sign when describing their pain, grasping the hip in the c-shape. Buttock pain and pain radiating down the posterior leg should alert the practitioner to the possibility of pathologic state of the lumbar spine. Pain in the lateral aspect of the hip may indicate trochanteric bursitis or iliotibial band friction syndrome. Pain that is strictly medial may indicate adductor muscle disease or hernias. Pain that presents superior to the inguinal ligament and radiates to the groin can be a presentation of a sports hernia or intra-abdominal, urologic, or gynecologic disease. The description of the pain can point the practitioner in a particular direction. Dull ache with intermittent sharp symptoms can represent any number of pathologic states. However, shooting or electric pain with numbness or tingling is often neurologic in origin.

The onset and provocation of the pain can often lead the practitioner to an appropriate diagnosis. Traumatic events should be carefully investigated in terms of the position of the leg at the time of the event and force directed

Conflict of Interest: We have no relevant conflict of interests to disclose with regard to this article and there was no funding received.

The Rothman Institute at Thomas Jefferson University Hospital, 925 Chestnut Street, 5th floor, Philadelphia, PA 19107, USA

* Corresponding author.

E-mail address: research@rothmaninstitute.com

Orthop Clin N Am 47 (2016) 485–496

http://dx.doi.org/10.1016/j.ocl.2016.03.002

against it because this will give clues to the structures and muscles involved. Frank dislocation of the native hip can also result in the late sequelae of avascular necrosis. Pain with deep flexion is characteristic of labral tears or chondrolabral junction injuries. These can also present with external rotation and extension. Participation in certain sports activities has been associated with particular injuries. Labral tears are more common in patients who participate in hockey, football, gymnastics, soccer, ballet, running, yoga, and surfing.[1,2] Runners are at high risk for iliotibial band friction syndrome and iliopsoas tendinitis. Mechanical symptoms indicate labral tears and chondral lesions. Painful clicking or snapping with flexion and extension is the presenting complaint of internal and external snapping hip (coxa saltans).

Medical History

Past medical history can give particular clues that should not be ignored, even in the young patient. A birth history indicating possible developmental dysplasia of the hip (DDH) should be elicited (even if the eventual diagnosis is made radiographically). First-borns, females, breech births, and oligohydramnios are the classic risk factors for DDH. It is important to know if patients had prior interventions for congenital hip dysplasia. A history of Legg-Calvé-Perthes or slipped capital femoral epiphysis may influence the choice of treatment and need for surgical intervention. A history of childhood obesity and endocrine disorders may raise suspicion for undiagnosed or subtle slipped capital femoral epiphysis. Any history with risk factors for avascular necrosis should be carefully teased out (eg, steroid use, alcohol, diving, human immunodeficiency virus infection [HIV], AIDS, antiretroviral therapy).

Physical Examination

The physical examination is a crucial portion of the diagnosis. The patient should first be observed ambulating. This exercise is most commonly done by watching the patient walk to the examination room before their knowledge of observation. Antalgic gait patterns should be observed carefully to help differentiate hip and knee disease. Knee or hip flexion contractures may also masquerade as antalgic gait. The practitioner should pay attention to foot progression angle as a clue for determining abnormal acetabular version. A Trendelenburg gait should be confirmed with the Trendelenburg sign and strength testing of the abductor muscles. Subtle abductor weakness can be present in patients

with DDH. Abductor muscle weakness also increases the joint reactive force and may exacerbate problems that might not otherwise cause patient discomfort. The subtleties of abnormal gait may help in specific diagnoses but may also identify deficiencies and targets for specified therapy. Studies have shown that patients with symptomatic FAI have lower voluntary motor contraction in all hip muscle groups (adduction, abduction, flexion, internal and external rotation) as well as lower electromyography (EMG) activity in certain muscles such as the tensor fasciae latae.[3] This can lead to specific kinematic and kinetic differences during gait. A study by Hunt and colleagues[4] compared 30 subjects with symptomatic FAI scheduled for surgery with 30 control subjects without FAI. They found that the subjects with FAI had a slower walking speed with slower cadence. Kinematically, the FAI group exhibited significantly less peak hip extension, adduction, and internal rotation during stance. Physical therapy targeting specific deficits may have a role in the treatment of patients with FAI, or comparative kinematic measurements may have a role in determining the success of the operative therapy. However, this has not been formally studied.

The patient should be examined standing as well as supine. Leg-length differences should be noted and compared with radiographs (full-length films should be obtained if there is any equivocation). Range of motion should be carefully tested and compared with the asymptomatic leg. During testing, attention must be paid during hip flexion and extension to detect flexion contractures. This can be done by having the patient flex both knees to the chest and then extend 1 knee at the time, thus removing lumbar compensation. The Stinchfield test (resisted hip flexion with the leg straight and 6 inches off the table) can help diagnose intra-articular problems because it indirectly loads the joint via muscle contraction. There are several tests for impingement, including flexion abduction external rotation (FABER) and flexion adduction internal rotation (FADIR). The extreme of flexion alone may cause impingement and symptoms may also be reproduced with hip external rotation and extension. The FABER test may also be positive with sacroiliitis. However, the location of this pain is usually over the sacroiliac joint and not in the groin, buttock, or lateral hip as with FAI. The Ober test helps determine iliotibial band tightness. Clear points of tenderness that lead to specific diagnoses include the bursa over the greater trochanter and over the iliotibial band insertion on Gerdy tubercle. Tenderness in the groin may represent iliopsoas disease, a hernia, or simply an inflamed hip capsule. A straight leg raise eliciting pain in the buttock (ipsilateral or contralateral) or reproducing radiating pain down the leg is highly suspicious for lumbar disease. Nerve tension signs, muscle strength, sensation, and reflexes should all be tested.

Differential Diagnosis

A logical and systematic approach is helpful in developing a differential diagnosis for hip pain. There are several schemas that may be useful. One is differential diagnosis by process as seen in Table 1. Another is differential diagnosis by anatomic location, as seen in Table 2.

Imaging

Imaging is of particular importance in reaching the correct diagnosis but certain pitfalls must be avoided. The correct interpretation of plain radiographs relies first and foremost on obtaining adequate films. Initial films include an anteroposterior (AP) pelvis with neutral rotation. When performed and interpreted adequately, this single view contains a wealth of information. The film should include the lower lumbar vertebrae as well as the proximal femora below the lesser trochanters. The practitioner should ensure that the film is neither an inlet nor an outlet view with the tip of the coccyx 3 to 4 cm from the pubic symphysis. On this view, the standard pelvic lines may be traced. A center-edge angle (CEA) and Tönnis angle can be calculated and crossover, posterior wall, and ischial spine signs observed for relative retroversion. The CEA of Wiberg (Fig. 1) is the angle formed between the 2 lines passing through the center of the femoral head, 1 of which extends to the lateral edge of sourcil and a line perpendicular to a horizontal line joining the centers of the 2 femoral heads (of the 2 hips). The normal Wiberg angle in an adult is greater than 25°. The CEA greater than 40° is usually considered abnormal

Table 1		
Group differential diagnosis of hip and groin pain		
Group	**Possible Diagnoses**	**Common Presentations**
Hip pain in the athlete	Muscle strains or tears, avulsions injuries, chondral or labral injuries, sports hernia	Often related to specific activities and movements or a single traumatic event
Congenital	Dysplasia	Insidious onset pain in the 2nd to 4th decade More common in females
Traumatic	Dislocation or subluxation, proximal femur fractures, chondral or labral injuries	Acute onset event
Vascular	Avascular necrosis	History of steroid use, alcohol, HIV Legg-Calvé-Perthes, leukemia, lymphoma, Gaucher, sickle cell, viral, lupus, hypercoagulable states, dysbaric disorders, irradiation, trauma
Metabolic	Transient osteoporosis	Middle-age men with no significant history, pregnant women
Inflammatory	Transient synovitis	Fever and groin pain relieved by NSAIDs Self-limited
Infection	Septic arthritis	Severe groin pain not relieved by NSAIDs
Impingement	FAI, labral tears	Pain with extremes of flexion, mechanical symptoms
Neoplastic	Synovial chondromatosis, PVNS	Groin pain and characteristic MRI appearance
Neurologic	Compression neuropathies and lumbar disease	Electric, shooting pain Pain in the buttock Numbness and tingling
Medications	As specific causes of AVN	Steroids, protease inhibitors

Abbreviations: AVN, atrioventricular node; NSAIDs, nonsteroidal antiinflammatory drugs; PVNS, pigmented villonodular synovitis.

Table 2
Location differential diagnosis of hip and groin pain

Intra-articular	Extra-articular Around the Hip	Pathologic Conditions Outside the Hip Joint
Labral tears	Trochanteric bursitis, Greater trochanteric pain syndrome	Lumbar radiculopathy
Chondral defects	Femoroischial impingement	Genitourinary (adnexa torsion, ectopic pregnancy, nephrolithiasis, orchitis, ovarian cysts, pelvic inflammatory disease, round ligament pain, round ligament torsion, urinary tract infection, endometriosis, prostatitis, testicular cancer)
FAI	Muscle injury (gluteal muscles, adductors, external rotators)	Intra-abdominal (abdominal aortic aneurysm, appendicitis, diverticulitis, lymphadenitis, diverticulosis, inflammatory bowel disease, inguinal or femoral hernia, tumors)
Capsular laxity	Piriformis syndrome	Sports hernia or athletic pubalgia
Ligamentum teres ruptures	Iliotibial band friction syndrome	Compression neuropathies (genitofemoral [L1, L2, L3], iliohypogastric [T12, L1], ilioinguinal [T12, L1], lateral femoral cutaneous [meralgia paresthetica], obturator, or pudendal)
Osteoarthritis	Iliopsoas tendinitis	
Inflammatory arthritis	Femoral stress fractures	
Osteonecrosis	Transient osteoporosis	
Loose bodies	Snapping hip (coxa saltans)	
Legg-Calvé-Perthes	Adductor strain	
Septic arthritis	Avulsion fractures	
SCFE	Iliofemoral ligament strain	
Synovitis	Sacroiliac injuries	
Instability	Pelvic stress fractures	
Synovial chondromatosis	Athletic pubalgia	
PVNS	Osteitis pubis	
Dysplasia	Psoas abscess	

Abbreviations: PVNS, pigmented villonodular synovitis; SCFE, slipped capital femoral epiphysis.

and may indicate pincer impingement. A CEA less than 25° indicates DDH. The Tönnis angle (Fig. 2) is formed by the intersection of a horizontal line connecting the femoral head centers and the line that passes through medial edge of the sourcil to its lateral edge. An angle of less than 0° may indicate impingement and an angle of greater than 10° may indicate dysplasia or instability. The crossover sign indicates acetabular retroversion and is determined when the shadow of the anterior wall crosses the shadow of the posterior wall. A hip with a normal pelvic inclination should have the anterior and posterior rims join at the edge of the acetabulum. A positive crossover sign is often accompanied by an ischial spine sign in which the ischial spine protrudes beyond the ilioischial line into the pelvis and is prominent. The posterior wall sign is positive when the posterior wall is medial to the center of the femoral head and

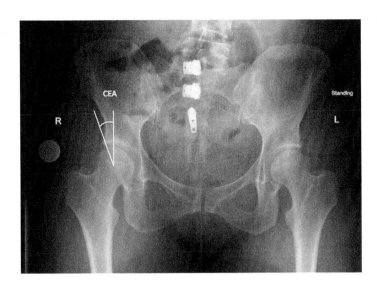

Fig. 1. CEA.

also indicates retroversion. Superior migration and extrusion of the femoral head are also notable signs of dysplasia and subtle changes can be detected by a break in Shenton line. The practitioner should look for signs of coxa profunda (fossa acetabuli touches or is medial to the ilioischial line) and protrusion acetabula (medial aspect of femoral head is medial to ilioischial line). A cross-table lateral is unreliable in determining acetabular version and the reader may also miss head-neck offset abnormalities. A frog-leg lateral may be useful in elucidating proximal femoral disease. A Dunn lateral view (flexion-abduction) is often used to better appreciate a cam lesion. The faux profile view can aid in evaluation of anterior coverage of the femoral head. On this view one can measure the anterior CEA in a similar fashion to measuring the lateral CEA on the AP radiograph. An anterior CEA less than 20° indicates a deficient anterior wall.

Advanced imaging is commonly performed in young patients with hip pain. Ultrasound can play a role in the diagnosis and management of certain tendinopathies, including tendinitis and tears of the abductors and iliopsoas, as well as trochanteric bursitis. Advanced cross-sectional imaging includes computed tomography (CT) and MRI, with or without intra-articular contrast. Further advanced imaging includes specialty MRI scans that examine the status of the articular cartilage, including T1-rho and delayed gadolinium-enhanced MRI of cartilage (dGEMRIC). MR arthrograms are

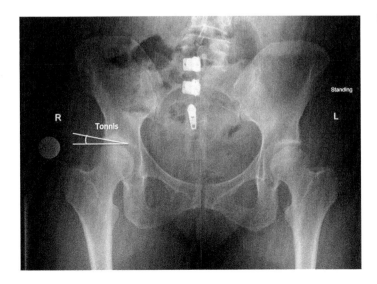

Fig. 2. Tönnis angle.

valuable tools for evaluating labral tears and chondral lesions with relatively high sensitivity and specificity but are limited by only fair inter-observer reliability as well as a lower reliability for detecting delaminated but not detached chondral lesions.[5–7] A study by Keeney and colleagues[7] examined 102 hips comparing MR arthrography with arthroscopic findings. In that study, magnetic resonance arthrography showed a sensitivity of 71%, specificity of 44%, positive predictive value of 93%, negative predictive value of 13%, and accuracy of 69% when evaluating labral disease. With respect to articular cartilage disease, MR arthrography had a sensitivity of 47%, specificity of 89%, positive predictive value of 84%, negative predictive value of 59%, and accuracy of 67%. A significant concern with MR arthrography, beyond the modest diagnostic accuracy, is the interpretation. Reurink and colleagues[6] compared 2 radiologists examining MR arthrograms of 95 hips scheduled for arthroscopy. They found a kappa of 0.268, indicating fair reliability at best. CT arthrography can also be used for assessment of the labrum and cartilage with high sensitivity and specificity but is less commonly used because it delivers a relatively high radiation dose.[8] Nishii and colleagues[8] reported on the use of isotropic high resolution CT arthrography in 20 hips compared with arthroscopic findings. With respect to labral tears, a sensitivity of 97%, specificity of 87%, and accuracy of 92% was found. For diagnosis of cartilage lesions, 88% sensitivity, 82% specificity, and 85% accuracy was reported.

With the aid of 3-T magnets, several MRI techniques have been developed that demonstrate the ability to examine cartilage quality. As the availability of 3-T MRI becomes more widespread, these techniques will likely become more commonly used in clinical practice. T2-MR mapping is able to distinguish between superficial and deep cartilage layers based on distribution of water relaxation times. Patients with hip dysplasia and normal radiographs have demonstrated high signal in the superficial layer using T2-mapping compared with healthy controls.[9] T1-rho MRI is a technique that is sensitive to low frequency chemical exchange between water molecules and the extracellular matrix of hyaline cartilage, revealing an inverse correlation between proteoglycan content and relaxation times. Rakhra and colleagues[10] compared 10 hips in symptomatic subjects with cam-type FAI to 10 controls. The control group demonstrated a T1-rho value trend, increasing from deep to superficial cartilage layers ($P = .008$). The FAI group demonstrated loss of this trend. The deepest third in the FAI group demonstrated greater T1-rho relaxation values than controls ($P = .028$). This suggests that the early cartilage changes in the FAI group not appreciated on normal MRI or plain radiographs can be teased out. Aside from clear applicability, the current downsides to T1-rho imaging include the specialized technology needed as well as the labor-intensive cartilage mapping required. Another recent, and more heavily studied, MRI development is dGEMRIC. The technique involves intravenous administration of gadolinium followed by a period of activity and subsequent MRI. The technique is sensitive to the charge density of glycosaminoglycans and has become a validated modality for detecting arthritis.[11,12] This imaging modality has established clinical utility. Studies have shown that the failure of pelvic osteotomies rises steeply in patients with a dGEMRIC index of less than 390 msec. This further supports the evidence that articular damage is poorly predictive of outcomes and this technology could become useful to develop more sensitive and specific cutoff values for hip preservation procedures than the current Tönnis grading system. The main downside to dGEMRIC is the intravenous administration of gadolinium and its inherent risk of nephrogenic systemic fibrosis or nephrogenic fibrosing dermopathy. Although many of the new imaging techniques are in their relative infancy regarding clinical utility, they hold promise for better patient selection and outcome measurement.

Aspiration or Injection

An intra-articular injection of a local anesthetic agent can provide both temporary pain relief and be a valuable diagnostic tool for differentiating from extra-articular causes of pain. Studies have shown injections to be safe and effective at reducing pain for up to 3 months in hip osteoarthritis, and the degree of relief has been correlated with the radiographic severity of arthritis. The efficacy of this intervention has not been fully studied in other diagnoses.[13,14] It is advisable for patients to keep a journal for the period surrounding the injection because the effectiveness of the injection has often decreased by the next clinic visit. Counseling younger patients without radiographic osteoarthritis of the purpose of this diagnostic tool can help avoid patient frustration with the outcome. Injections can also be directed into the iliopsoas tendon sheath or trochanteric bursa and can provide significant pain relief. If infection is suspected, aspiration is a crucial part of diagnosis but should not delay treatment in the native hip. Both aspiration and injection should be performed by a qualified practitioner under radiographic or ultrasound guidance.

Extra Tests

EMG and nerve conduction studies can be helpful in differentiating nerve compression syndromes and radiculopathy. Unfortunately, certain muscles groups around the hip are difficult to test due to their depth in the soft tissue.

Treatment Options

The treatment options for all possible conditions affecting the hip is beyond the scope of this article. Instead, the focus is on anatomic disease with possible surgical interventions. Labral tears, FAI, and dysplasia often lie on a spectrum of severity, and associated pathologic states should be carefully weighed before treatment ensues.

Nonoperative Management

The treatment of many conditions affecting the hip of a young patient should begin with nonoperative management. The initial nonoperative measures include activity modification, administration of nonopioid analgesics and topical anesthetics, anti-inflammatories, physical therapy, chiropractic or osteopathic therapy, weight loss, and injections. Overall, the quality of evidence for nonoperative management is low. A meta-analysis of 53 papers examining nonoperative treatment of FAI found only 5 papers with any experimental analysis. All of these were small case series or descriptive epidemiologic studies of low or very low quality. Several similarities were found in the studies that may aid in advising patients. First, nonoperative management may improve symptoms in certain patients. Second, attempts to improve passive or active range of motion may be counterproductive given the mechanical nature of the deformity.[15] Overall, there is little harm in attempting a course of nonoperative management with therapy and counseling regarding activity modification. Short-term use of anti-inflammatories may be helpful to progress the patient through a difficult period of symptoms. Long-term use of anti-inflammatories includes significant risks such as gastrointestinal distress, bleeding, myocardial infarction, and stroke, and should be pursued with caution.

Labral Tears

Which labral tears are most amenable to repair remains a matter of controversy. Careful diagnostic evaluation includes appropriate imaging, and intra-articular injection should be strongly considered before treatment. A long trial of nonoperative management should be the norm before any surgical intervention. If surgical intervention is deemed necessary, the surgeon should carefully address the labral tear and any underlying anatomic abnormality that could lead to recurrence. There is no consensus regarding arthroscopic versus open repairs. Proponents of the arthroscopic approach note the ability to visualize the central compartment and small, minimally invasive incisions. There is no literature comparing outcomes between arthroscopic in the supine or lateral decubitus positions. Despite being minimally invasive, there are significant risks, including neurovascular injury either from the instruments or traction. Ankle fractures from the positioning boot are another known risk. Arthroscopically assisted, mini-open procedures have been described without the use of a traction table. Advantages to the open approach include a relatively small incision that can be extended for hip arthroplasty or periacetabular osteotomy (PAO), a relatively short procedure time, lack of need for a specialized table, and avoidance of traction. Both arthroscopic and mini-open procedures allow for visualization and repair of the labrum, as well as the ability to address osseous lesions involved in FAI. However, both procedures are limited in their ability to address posterior lesions.

Over the last decade, there has been an increasingly large body of literature regarding the treatment of labral tears. Almost all studies are low-grade evidence in case series, prospective cohorts, and small randomized controlled trials. However, outcomes have been good in carefully selected subjects. A review of literature by Robertson and colleagues[16] found a patient satisfaction rate of 67% at 3.5 years with 50% relief of mechanical symptoms. There is some evidence that repair of the labrum is a better option than debridement. A systematic review of the treatment of labral tears during surgery for FAI looked specifically at debridement versus repair. The investigators found a significant improvement in patient outcomes in the modified Harris hip score of 7.4 points favoring repair.[17] It is also critical to recognize that up to 90% of patients with labral tears have an underlying structural abnormality.

Femoroacetabular Impingement

FAI is defined as abnormal femoral and/or acetabular morphology resulting in adherent contact between the 2 surfaces. As a result, there is supraphysiologic motion and repetitive loading that leads to soft tissue damage. The entity is typically grouped into cam, pincer, or combined cam-type and pincer-type. Usually pain presents in the groin, radiating laterally toward the greater trochanter and medially toward the adductors. Symptoms may rarely radiate to the buttock and down to the medial knee. Pain is often positional and exacerbated by flexion or prolonged sitting. There is a distinct loss of motion of the hip, particularly in flexion, abduction, and internal rotation. Imaging signs consistent with FAI include a crossover sign, ischial spine sign, increased CEA, increased alpha-angle on CT or Dunn radiograph, and small cysts at the femoral head neck junction (ie, herniation pits). Labral tears and cartilage delamination can occur as a result of FAI. Another distinct, although rare, impingement entity is femoral-ischial impingement and the practitioner should be aware of patients with extremely low offset.

Whether or not FAI is a prearthritic condition or a reaction to an arthritic process remains a debate. Ganz and colleagues[18] have championed that greater than 90% of hip osteoarthritis may be attributable to pre-existing deformity. However, cross-sectional and epidemiologic studies create some doubt in this claim by revealing morphologic abnormalities in a large, asymptomatic portion of the population.[19]

Treatment of FAI has shown relatively good results in a carefully selected population who have Tönnis grade 0 or 1 osteoarthrosis. Arthroscopy allows access for treatment of anterior cam lesions and labral repairs. There is increased difficulty in addressing acetabular lesions, cartilage damage, or impingement in the inferior and posterior aspects of the hip. Additionally, neurovascular risks from instruments and prolonged traction are disadvantages of this intervention. The mini-open option via 4 cm modified Smith-Peterson approach can address both femoral and acetabular lesions without difficulty, does not require a special table or traction, and has a relatively quick recovery. However, there is a limitation in the access to posterior lesions as well as the central compartment. Surgical hip dislocation with a trochanteric osteotomy can address the full spectrum of femoral and acetabular pathologic conditions with good results but is associated with significant surgical morbidity. If the patient has acetabular retroversion and concomitant cam-type FAI, then a PAO should be considered. For the patient with posterior impingement and excessive posterior wall coverage, a reverse PAO is an option but outcomes have been variable.

Overall outcomes from treatment of FAI are generally good with arthroscopic, mini-open procedures, or surgical hip dislocations. Literature reviews show that, overall, 75% to 90% of athletes return to sport at their preinjury level. Reduced pain and improvement of function are reported in 68% to 96% of patients with an improvement range of 2.4 to 5 points on the Merle d'Aubigné and Postel score.[20] The heterogeneity of outcomes and lack of positive outcomes in some studies can be partially explained by the consistent findings that patients with pre-existing arthritis, advanced chondral degeneration, and older age had worse outcomes with faster progression to total hip replacement.[21,22] This finding confirms that conservative patient selection is critical for success when considering hip preservation.

Cartilage Lesions

Most cartilage lesions are associated with labral tears and often with FAI or dysplasia.[23] Major cartilage lesions are usually best treated with arthroplasty. However, other options exist, including chondroplasty, microfracture, articular cartilage repair or reattachment, autologous chondrocyte implantation (ACI), mosaicplasty, and osteochondral allograft transplantation (OAT). Most of these techniques are well described in the knee but outcomes in the hip are less reported. Microfracture is described for contained lesions less than 4 cm^2, and several case series have been published with generally favorable results.[24,25] Byrd and Jones[26] reported on microfracture during management of FAI in 58 hips with a grade 4 chondral defect, an intact subchondral plate, and healthy surrounding cartilage. The modified Harris hip score improved from 65 preoperatively to 85 at 2-year follow-up. The relative advantages of microfracture over other cartilage procedures are low expense and ease of performing. The durability of the subsequent fibrocartilage repair is unknown. ACI is performed in a staged manner in which chondrocytes are harvested from 1 joint, grown in a laboratory, and then reimplanted using a patch or with matrix-assisted ACI (MACI). Fontana and colleagues[27] compared the outcomes of simple debridement versus MACI for management of hip chondral defects in 30 subjects with Outerbridge grade 3 or 4 lesions. The area of the defect was equal in both groups, as was the preoperative Harris hip score, with 48.3 in the MACI group and 46 in the debridement group. The investigators reported better clinical outcomes with MACI than with simple chondroplasty, with an average

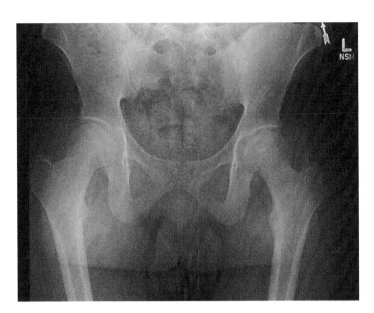

Fig. 3. Preoperative radiograph of an 18-year-old patient with symptomatic right hip dysplasia.

Harris hip score of 87.4 in the MACI group and an average score of 56.3 in the debridement group (P<.05) at final follow-up. Mosaicplasty is the use of cylindrical cartilage plugs with subchondral bone attached to fill defects of large size. The technique has been well described in the knee but only small case series have been reported in the hip with good results. Girard and colleagues[28] reported 10 subjects with femora head defects and an average age of 18 years with a variety of congenital hip diseases. Average lesion size was 4.8 cm² and the average follow-up was 29.2 months. The Merle d'Aubigné and Postel score improved from an average of 10.5 preoperatively to an average of 15.5 postoperatively. The Harris hip score also improved from 52.8 preoperatively to 79.5 postoperatively. At 6 months postoperatively, CT arthrograms showed excellent graft incorporation with intact cartilage in all subjects. At final follow-up, none of the subjects required total hip arthroplasty (THA). The downsides to the procedure include donor site morbidity and the necessity for surgical hip dislocation. An OAT procedure may be appropriate for larger defects with subchondral bone loss. An early study by Meyers and colleagues[29] had a 32% failure rate (8 out of 25 hips). More recently, Khanna and colleagues[30] reported good outcomes in 76% of subjects (13 out of 17 hips). Failures, durability, and risk of disease transmission are the major concerns regarding OAT procedures. Overall, larger, high quality studies are needed to delineate the appropriate patients and lesions for cartilage restoration.

Dysplasia

There is a spectrum of abnormal hip morphology under the umbrella term of congenital hip dysplasia. This includes acetabular version, depth and coverage, proximal femoral deformities, and their combined resultant altered biomechanics and pathologic states. The spectrum can cause pain and labral disease either through too little bone, as seen in the undercoverage and anteversion of classic dysplasia, or too much bone, as seen in coxa profunda, the cam, and pincer FAI. Treatment of these morphologies in the prearthritic hip of the younger patient includes a variety of acetabular and

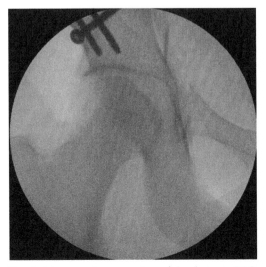

Fig. 4. Intraoperative correction of dysplasia via PAO.

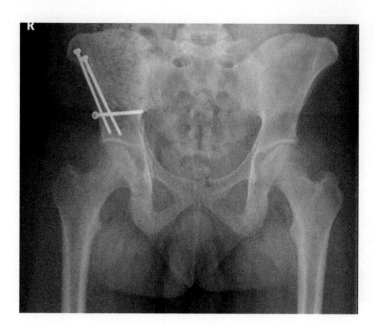

Fig. 5. Postoperative radiograph demonstrating healed PAO and excellent correction of dysplasia.

proximal femoral osteotomies, combined with treatment of any underlying labral disease, and FAI. When indicated, a Bernese PAO can be combined with a femoral osteoplasty and labral repair through a single direct anterior incision (Figs. 3–5). Certain femoral deformities may require a proximal femoral osteotomy. In general, these are complex procedures that require specialized training and have relatively high complication rates. A systematic review revealed a major complication rate of 6% to 37%, including symptomatic heterotopic ossification, major nerve injuries, intra-articular osteotomies, loss of fixation, and malreduction.[31]

The PAO has become a widely accepted surgical procedure for hip dysplasia with mid-term and long-term results available. The original outcomes published by Ganz and colleagues[32] in 1988 were re-examined in 2008 by Steppacher and colleagues[33] with a minimum of 19-year follow-up. They were able to follow up on 68 of 75 hips. Of these, 60% were preserved at final follow-up corresponding to a Kaplan-Meier survivorship of 60.5%. The overall Merle d'Aubigné and Postel score decreased compared with the 10-year values and had become similar to preoperative scores. As practitioners have become more experienced with the PAO and patient selection has improved, mid-term outcomes have become similar to total hip replacement. Gray and colleagues[34] reported on 2 consecutive cohorts comparing PAO and THA. They included subjects between aged 18 to 40 years who had undergone either PAO (100 hips; 24 male

subjects, 76 female subjects) or THA (55 hips; 18 male subjects, 37 female subjects). At a mean follow-up of 5.9 years (2–13), there was a statistically significant improvement in the modified Harris hip pain, function, and total scores within each cohort with no significant differences in scores between the groups. For subjects with Tönnis grade 0 or 1, the PAO has been shown to be a pain relieving and cost-effective intervention.[35]

SUMMARY OR DISCUSSION

Hip pain in the young adult can be a challenging problem requiring a systematic approach to the patient. Management of intra-articular, anatomic, and mechanical problems including FAI, dysplasia, labral tears, and cartilage injury is evolving but good treatment options exist. There is very little evidence regarding the natural evolution of labral tears, FAI, and dysplasia with nonoperative management. Further research is necessary to better delineate appropriate patient selection for hip preservation and to develop improved indications and techniques for cartilage restoration. Surgical management with hip preservation procedures in carefully selected patients can have excellent outcomes.

REFERENCES

1. Frank JS, Gambacorta PL, Eisner EA. Hip pathology in the adolescent athlete. J Am Acad Orthop Surg 2013;21:665–74.

2. Wilson JJ, Furukawa M. Evaluation of the patient with hip pain. Am Fam Physician 2014;89:27–34.

3. Casartelli NC, Maffiuletti NA, Item-Glatthorn JF, et al. Hip muscle weakness in patients with symptomatic femoroacetabular impingement. Osteoarthr Cartil 2011;19:816–21.

4. Hunt MA, Gunether JR, Gilbart MK. Kinematic and kinetic differences during walking in patients with and without symptomatic femoroacetabular impingement. Clin Biomech 2013;28:519–23.

5. Leunig M, Podeszwa D, Beck M, et al. Magnetic resonance arthrography of labral disorders in hips with dysplasia and impingement. Clin Orthop Relat Res 2004;(418):74–80.

6. Reurink G, Jansen SPL, Bisselink JM, et al. Reliability and validity of diagnosing acetabular labral lesions with magnetic resonance arthrography. J Bone Joint Surg Am 2012;94:1643–8.

7. Keeney JA, Peelle MW, Jackson J, et al. Magnetic resonance arthrography versus arthroscopy in the evaluation of articular hip pathology. Clin Orthop Relat Res 2004;429:163–9.

8. Nishii T, Tanaka H, Sugano N, et al. Disorders of acetabular labrum and articular cartilage in hip dysplasia: evaluation using isotropic high-resolutional CT arthrography with sequential radial reformation. Osteoarthr Cartil 2007;15:251–7.

9. Nishii T, Tanaka H, Sugano N, et al. Evaluation of cartilage matrix disorders by T2 relaxation time in patients with hip dysplasia. Osteoarthr Cartil 2008;16:227–33.

10. Rakhra KS, Lattanzio P-J, Cardenas-Blanco A. Can T1-rho MRI detect acetabular cartilage degeneration in femoroacetabular impingement?: A pilot study. J Bone Jt Surg - Br Vol 2012;94-B:1187–92.

11. Kim Y-J, Jaramillo D, Millis MB, et al. Assessment of early osteoarthritis in hip dysplasia with delayed gadolinium-enhanced magnetic resonance imaging of cartilage. J Bone Joint Surg Am 2003;85A:1987–92.

12. Chandrasekaran S, Vemula SP, Lindner D, et al. Preoperative delayed gadolinium-enhanced magnetic resonance imaging of cartilage (dGEMRIC) for patients undergoing hip arthroscopy. J Bone Joint Surg Am 2015;97(16):1305–15.

13. Hirsch G, Kitas G, Klocke R. Intra-articular corticosteroid injection in osteoarthritis of the knee and hip: factors predicting pain relief-a systematic review. Semin Arthritis Rheum 2013;42:451–73.

14. Deshmukh AJ, Panagopoulos G, Alizadeh A, et al. Intra-articular hip injection: does pain relief correlate with radiographic severity of osteoarthritis? Skeletal Radiol 2011;40:1449–54.

15. Wall PDH, Fernandez M, Griffin DR, et al. Nonoperative treatment for femoroacetabular impingement: a systematic review of the literature. PM R 2013;5:418–26.

16. Robertson WJ, Kadrmas WR, Kelly BT. Arthroscopic management of labral tears in the hip: a systematic review of the literature. Clin Orthop Relat Res 2007;455:88–92.

17. Ayeni OR, Adamich J, Farrokhyar F, et al. Surgical management of labral tears during femoroacetabular impingement surgery: a systematic review. Knee Surg Sports Traumatol Arthrosc 2014;22:756–62.

18. Ganz R, Leunig M, Leunig-Ganz K, et al. The etiology of osteoarthritis of the hip: an integrated mechanical concept. Clin Orthop Relat Res 2008;466:264–72.

19. Sankar WN, Nevitt M, Parvizi J, et al. Femoroacetabular impingement: defining the condition and its role in the pathophysiology of osteoarthritis. J Am Acad Orthop Surg 2013;21(Suppl 1):S7–15.

20. Bedi A, Kelly BT. Femoroacetabular impingement. J Bone Joint Surg Am 2013;95:82–92.

21. Clohisy JC, St John LC, Schutz AL. Surgical treatment of femoroacetabular impingement: a systematic review of the literature. Clin Orthop Relat Res 2010;468:555–64.

22. Ng VY, Arora N, Best TM, et al. Efficacy of surgery for femoroacetabular impingement: a systematic review. Am J Sports Med 2010;38:2337–45.

23. McCarthy JC, Lee J-A. Arthroscopic intervention in early hip disease. Clin Orthop Relat Res 2004;(429):157–62.

24. Macdonald AE, Bedi A, Horner NS, et al. Indications and outcomes for microfracture as an chondral defects in patients with femoroacetabular. Arthroscopy 2016;32(1):190–200.e2.

25. El Bitar YF, Lindner D, Jackson TJ, et al. Joint-preserving Surgical Options for Management of Chondral Injuries of the Hip. J Am Acad Orthop Surg 2014;22:46–56.

26. Byrd JWT, Jones KS. Arthroscopic femoroplasty in the management of cam-type femoroacetabular impingement. Clin Orthop Relat Res 2009;467:739–46.

27. Fontana A, Bistolfi A, Crova M, et al. Arthroscopic treatment of hip chondral defects: autologous chondrocyte transplantation versus simple debridement–a pilot study. Arthroscopy 2012;28:322–9.

28. Girard J, Roumazeille T, Sakr M, et al. Osteochondral mosaicplasty of the femoral head. Hip Int 2011;21:542–8.

29. Meyers MH, Jones RE, Bucholz RW, et al. Fresh autogenous grafts and osteochondral allografts for the treatment of segmental collapse in osteonecrosis of the hip. Clin Orthop Relat Res 1983;(174):107–12.

30. Khanna V, Tushinski DM, Drexler M, et al. Cartilage restoration of the hip using fresh osteochondral allograft: resurfacing the potholes. Bone Joint J 2014;96B:11–6.

31. Clohisy JC, Schutz AL, St John L, et al. Periacetabular osteotomy: a systematic literature review. Clin Orthop Relat Res 2009;467:2041–52.

32. Ganz R, Klaue K, Vinh TS, et al. A new periacetabular osteotomy for the treatment of hip dysplasias. Technique and preliminary results. Clin Orthop Relat Res 1988;(232):26–36.

33. Steppacher SD, Tannast M, Ganz R, et al. Mean 20-year followup of Bernese periacetabular osteotomy. Clin Orthop Relat Res 2008;466:1633–44.

34. Gray BL, Stambough JB, Schoenecker PL. Comparison of contemporary periacetabular osteotomy for hip dysplasia with total hip arthroplasty for hip osteoarthritis. Bone Joint J 2015;97B(10):1322–7.

35. Sharifi E, Sharifi H, Morshed S, et al. Cost-effectiveness analysis of periacetabular osteotomy. J Bone Joint Surg Am 2008;90:1447–56.

Total Hip Arthroplasty Performed Through Direct Anterior Approach Provides Superior Early Outcome

Results of a Randomized, Prospective Study

Javad Parvizi, MD, FRCS*, Camilo Restrepo, MD,
Mitchell G. Maltenfort, PhD, MBA

KEYWORDS

• Total hip • Direct anterior approach • Direct lateral approach • Outcomes • Complications

KEY POINTS

- Total hip arthroplasty (THA) performed through the direct anterior (DA) approach provides better early functional outcomes as measured by the validated functional instruments. These patients are able to return to work and gain functional independence earlier than their counterparts who receive surgery through the direct lateral approach and are subjected to the same postoperative rehabilitation protocols.
- The use of the DA approach, and the lack of need for muscle strengthening, reduces the need for physical therapy following discharge from the hospital. This difference minimizes cost, enhances functional recovery, and allows early return to driving and work.
- Performing THA through a DA approach, particularly without the proper training, may be challenging for the first few cases. Thus, there is a certain level of learning involved with this surgical approach. It is therefore paramount that surgeons unfamiliar with this approach who wish to adopt the DA approach for THA need to subject themselves to extensive cadaveric training.

INTRODUCTION

In recent years total hip arthroplasty (THA) performed through the direct anterior (DA) approach using the Hueter interval has been gaining popularity. This approach uses an internervous and intermuscular access to the hip joint and avoids violation of the abductor muscles or short rotators around the hip. Because of its minimally invasive nature, patients are expected to have a better early functional outcome, at least once the surgeon is beyond the learning curve.[1–6] Numerous level 1 studies have compared the outcomes of THA performed through the DA approach with those of patients receiving THA either through direct lateral (DL) approach or posterolateral approach. In all of these studies, THA performed through the DA approach had better early functional outcome. In addition, patients receiving THA through the DA approach reported returning to daily activities, such as driving, more quickly.[6–8]

Although based on available evidence, early outcomes of THA performed through the DA

Source of Funding: Zimmer provided financial support for this study.

The Rothman Institute at Thomas Jefferson University Hospital, 925 Chestnut Street, Philadelphia, PA 19107, USA

* Corresponding author.

E-mail address: research@rothmaninstitute.com

http://dx.doi.org/10.1016/j.ocl.2016.03.003
0030-5898/16/$ – see front matter

approach are superior to THA performed through other approaches, but a few facts still remain unknown.[6] It is not known whether the superior outcome of THA performed through the DA approach applies to the very early time period, (ie, within hours). It is also not known by what time point in the postoperative period the functional outcome of THA done through other approaches catches up with the patients who undergo THA through a DA approach. This article addresses both of these questions and discusses a randomized, prospective study with specific objectives.

MATERIAL AND METHODS

Following institutional review board approval, all patients with end-stage arthritis of the hip needing THA were approached and consented to participate in this randomized, prospective study. The study was also enlisted in http://www.clinicaltrials.gov. Randomization was performed using a random number generator in an electronic spread sheet. Patients were assigned to 1 of 2 groups. One group of patients received THA using the DA approach (modified Smith-Petersen), whereas others were assigned to receive THA using the DL approach (modified Hardinge) (Fig. 1). The study began in February 2012 and enrollment completed in November 2013. During the period of study, 75 patients (84 hips) were recruited into the study. Throughout the same period, 47 other patients were also approached for enrollment but declined to be part of the study. The responses that eliminated participation included preference of a surgical approach (8 patients), unwillingness to participate in the follow-up data collection (3 patients), and not specifically providing a reason (36 patients). All patients

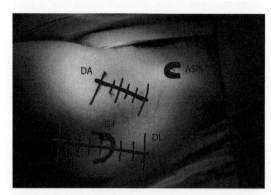

Fig. 1. The anatomic landmarks of the DA and DL incisions. ASIS, anterior superior ischial spine; GT, greater trochanter.

undergoing conversion THA, revision THA, or complex THA that required an additional surgical approach or exposure, such as trochanteric slide or osteotomy, were also excluded.

In addition, and as a requirement of the institutional review board, the patients needed to be between the ages of 18 and 75 years, have the underlying diagnosis of osteoarthritis, able to read and comprehend English, and to sign the consent form to participate in the study. Patients with cognitive impairment or severe psychiatric illness that would preclude participation in the protocol mandated procedures were excluded. The purpose of the study and the method, including the randomization, were discussed in detail with the patients before the consent was obtained. The patients were informed that they would receive 1 of 2 surgical approaches, both of which were safe and effective. The risks of the surgical procedure were also discussed in detail with the patients.

All patients were subjected to the same preoperative and postoperative protocols for rehabilitation, pain management, and anticoagulation. There were 18 men (40.9%) and 26 (59.1%) women in the DA group, compared with 14 (35.0%) men and 26 (65%) women in the DL group.

Preoperative Protocol
The patients were evaluated in the outpatient setting. Patients were told they would be subjected to THA using either the DA or the DL approach. Patients were not advised that one was likely to provide better early outcomes than the other. The postoperative analgesia protocol was also discussed in detail; patients were told it would include oral opioid and nonopioid analgesics supplemented by intravenous medications, if needed. The patients were reassured that their pain would be well controlled. The patients were told about the benefits of early ambulation and encouraged to comply with the rehabilitation protocol, which involved assisted ambulation on the day of surgery and twice daily thereafter. Patients were told that home discharge was preferred and family members were encouraged to care for the patient at home.

Surgical Data
All patients received spinal anesthesia using 0.2 mg of DepoMorphine. Intravenous propofol, midazolam, and opioid analgesics such as morphine, fentanyl, or meperidine were administered at the discretion of the anesthesiologist.

A detailed record of all intraoperative analgesics was maintained.

The surgery was performed in supine position on a regular operating table that could be flexed at the hip for the DA patients. The initial incision length was 5 cm, and the incision was lengthened as dictated by the need for surgical exposure. The only difference between the two groups was the location of the incision, which was placed laterally over the greater trochanter for the DL patients, and more anteriorly for the DA patients. The DA approach involved exposure of tensor fascia lata and division of its perimysium. The interval between sartorius and tensor fascia lata was not used in order to minimize the risk of injury to the lateral femoral cutaneous nerve. The lateral head or reflected portion of rectus was not incised but was retracted medially. Anterior capsulotomy was performed, preserving the capsule for later closure, and the femoral neck was exposed. A double osteotomy of the neck was performed and a wedge of bone from the femoral neck was removed to allow easy extraction of the remaining head. The preparation of the acetabulum and the femoral canal was then performed in the routine manner. Exposure of the femoral canal involved selected soft tissue releases on the posterior aspect of the femoral neck ensuring that the abductor mechanism and the short rotators of the hip were preserved. Modified instruments for the exposure of acetabulum and the femur were used during the DA approach, which included the use of a double offset broach handle for the femur.

The DL approach was performed by placement of the incision over the greater trochanter and division of the underlying fascia lata. The abductor mechanism was divided and the anterior one-half retracted anteriorly. Following capsulotomy, the hip was dislocated and the femoral neck was cut. Acetabular and femoral preparation was conducted in a conventional manner.

Uncemented femoral and acetabular components were used in all patients, which included a proximally coated, collarless, tapered femoral stem (ML Taper, Zimmer, Warsaw, IN) and a porous tantalum acetabular component (Continuum, Zimmer, Warsaw, IN). The type of bearing surface used was delta ceramic femoral head and highly cross-linked polyethylene (Longevity, Zimmer, Warsaw, IN) in all patients.

All surgical parameters, including estimated blood loss, operative time, intraoperative complications, and any other pertinent information, were recorded in detail. A full-time clinical coordinator was assigned to this study.

Postoperative Management

Appropriate prophylaxis for infection (Ancef [GlaxoSmithKline LLC, Middlesex, United Kingdom] preoperatively and for 24 hours postoperatively), and thromboembolism (aspirin [Bayer, Leverkusen, Germany] 81 mg twice a day for 4 weeks) was administered to all the patients according to our protocols.

Blood management included administration of 1 g of tranexamic acid intravenously before incision to all patients. Allogeneic blood transfusion was provided when necessary. Hemodynamic symptoms triggering transfusion included persistent tachycardia (heart rate >100 beats/min for at least 4 hours) and lassitude (inability to comply with physical therapy exercises). Any patients with dyspnea or chest pain were extensively evaluated. The internal medicine specialists, unaware of the status of the patients in the study, were responsible for hemoglobin management. The details of blood transfusion were recorded.

All patients received a social service consultant, who was also blinded to the surgical approach. The purpose was to discuss social circumstances and confirm the preoperatively determined disposition plan based on the degree of home support, the home layout, and the patient's physical abilities. On occasions, patients initially assumed to be candidates for home discharge were sent to a skilled rehabilitation facility at the recommendation of the physical therapy team.

The cumulative dose and the type of analgesic medications administered during hospital stay were recorded in detail for each patient. The equianalgesic dose for all drugs was calculated. The equianalgesic conversion based on pain-relieving efficacy equivalent to 10 mg of morphine was used. Patients were placed initially on oral opioid medication (oxycodone 5 mg every 4 to 6 hours as needed) and oral nonopioid analgesics such as ketorolac were administered based on each patient's needs and level of pain.

The patients were seen by a physical therapist a few hours after arrival on the ward and helped to sit in a chair or ambulate with assistance, if possible. Physical therapy occurred at least twice daily thereafter. The wounds were covered by a single occlusive dressing, which was kept in place for 5 to 7 days. The physical therapists were kept unaware of the type of approach that each patient had received.

Functional Outcome

The functional outcomes on day 1, day 2, week 6, week 12, 6 months, and 1 year were measured using the time-to-get-up-and-go (TUG), gait speed, chair test,[9] Linear Analogue Scale (LASA),[10] Harris Hip Score (HHS),[9,11] and Lower Extremity Functional Score (LEFS).[12] These tests included a timed test involving the patient standing from a seated position in a chair and walking 10 feet before turning around and returning to a seated position in the same chair without stopping (TUG). Gait speed is a timed test in which a patient walks a premeasured distance and velocity is measured. The chair test records the time required for a patient to stand from a seated position in a chair 5 consecutive times without the use of armrests for support. In addition, patients' Functional Independence Measure subscores were recorded, which included patients' locomotion status (complete independence, modified independence, supervision, minimal assistance, moderate assistance, maximal assistance, and total assistance), walking distance, the type of walking aid used (single-point cane, axillary crutches, rolling walker, or standard walker), return to work, and return to driving.

Follow-up

On discharge, patients were instructed to complete a daily diary that attempted to capture their functional recovery and analgesia consumption. A strict follow-up protocol was followed to closely monitor the patients recruited into this study. All patients were seen in the office and examined by an independent observer as well as the senior surgeon at or around 4 weeks postoperatively. Patients were then followed at routine intervals, which included a visit at 6 months, 1 year, and then at 2 years. Clinical examination and radiographic evaluation were performed during the follow-up. The independent blinded observer collected the data on all patients.

Statistical Analysis

Before initiation of the study a power analysis was performed by a statistician to ensure enrollment of an adequate sample size. For an effect size of 20% with alpha set to 0.05 and a power of 0.80, 40 patients were needed in each group. In addition to the required 80 subjects, 10 more patients in each group were recruited to allow for possible attrition.

Baseline and information collected at each study visit were compared between each intervention group using the Wilcoxon test for continuous variables and Fisher exact test for binary outcomes. Longitudinal analysis of outcomes was performed using a linear mixed effects model. All analyses were performed using R.3.1 (R Foundation for Statistical Computing, Vienna, Austria).

RESULTS

Functional Outcome

There was a significant improvement in function as measured by the HHS, the LASA, the TUG, the gait speed test, and the LEFS, following THA in both groups. The functional outcomes were the same for both groups at the latest follow-up at 1 year. However, there was a significant difference in some aspects of functional outcome at the early time points (both before and at 6 weeks, at 6 months, and even at 1 year postoperative) between the two groups, with DA patients having a better function in the TUG ($P = .0001$) (Fig. 2), gait speed ($P = .0001$) (Fig. 3), and LEFS ($P = .0267$) (Fig. 4). Patients undergoing THA using the DA approach were able to return to work ($P<.08$) and able to drive ($P<.002$) earlier than their counterparts who received surgery through the DL approach (Fig. 5).

Other Outcomes

There was no difference in operative time ($P = .3068$), the estimated blood loss ($P = .669$), decrease in hemoglobin level ($P = .440$), need for transfusion ($P = .692$), and length of hospital stay ($P = .562$) between the two groups (Table 1).

Few orthopedic complications were encountered in this cohort, including 1 dislocation, 1 irrigation and debridement for persistent wound drainage, and 1 nondisplaced proximal femoral fracture. One patient with severe bronchitis was hospitalized.

DISCUSSION

This randomized prospective study shows that THA performed through the DA approach provides better early functional outcome as measured by the validated functional instruments. In addition, these patients were able to return to work and gain functional independence earlier than their counterparts who received surgery through the DL approach and were subjected to the same postoperative rehabilitation protocols. We were not able to detect any difference in analgesia consumption, blood transfusion, or hospital length of stay between the two groups. The reason for the length of stay may relate to the strict care protocols, such as administration of tranexamic acid for blood management and fast track rehabilitation.

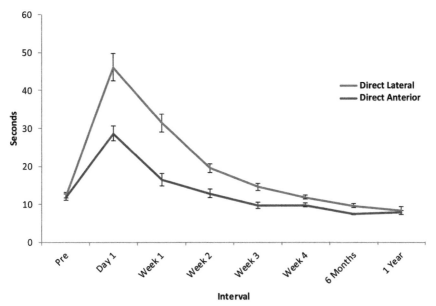

Fig. 2. Comparison between DL and DA functional outcomes using the TUG test.

All patients in this study received spinal anesthesia and multimodal pain management. Patients are also allowed and encouraged to leave the hospital on postoperative day 1. Under these circumstances, and with the given sample size, it is not surprising that no significant difference in some of these parameters was observed.

These findings are in line with many prior level 1 comparative studies that have evaluated the outcome of THA performed through the DA approach.[1–6,13] The objective of this study was to evaluate the very early outcome of THA in these two groups. With the ever-increasing demand on THA and limited resources that are available, there is a great pressure to provide a high level of care and allow early return of patients to full function.[14] The improvements in anesthesia techniques, pain management, rehabilitation, and blood management have allowed orthopedic surgeons to accomplish great advances in total joint arthroplasty. The use of a minimally invasive and true inter-nervous plane of dissection is one such advance because surgeons avoid detachment of any musculature.

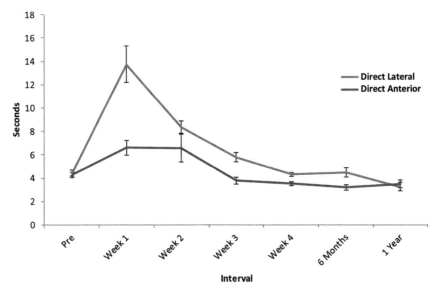

Fig. 3. Comparison between DL and DA functional outcome gate speed.

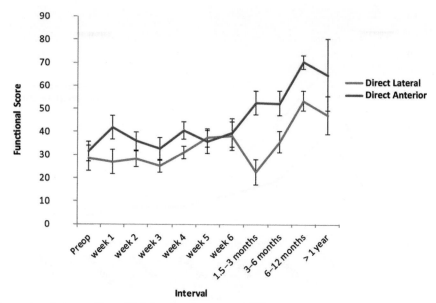

Fig. 4. Comparison between DL and DA functional outcome LEFS.

However, any advances in surgery have come at a cost. Performing THA through a DA approach, particularly without the proper training, may be challenging for the first few cases. There is a learning curve associated with this surgical approach.[4] It is highly recommended that surgeons unfamiliar with this approach participate in educational activities such as cadaveric training. In addition, surgeons should perform this procedure selectively on patients with low body mass index and uncomplicated anatomy during their learning curve in an attempt to minimize complications.[15] The senior surgeon in this study has been performing THA using both of

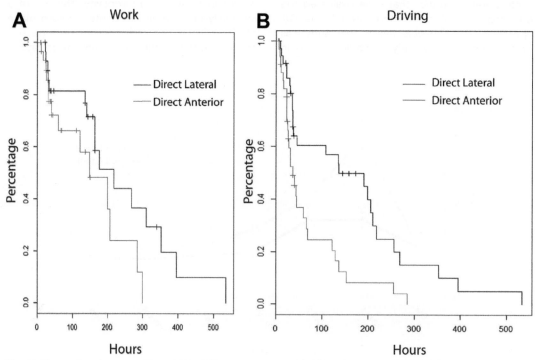

Fig. 5. Comparison between DL and DA ability to return to work (A) and return to driving (B).

Table 1
Other outcomes measured in between both groups

	DL	DA	P-value
Operative time in minutes (range)	87.53 (53–241)	84.51 (51–185)	.3068
EBL in milliliters (range)	257.40 (100–600)	209 (50–750)	.6690
Hematocrit percentage decrease (range)	9.5 (3.5–14)	10.7 (5.5–16.4)	.4400
LOS in hours (range)	36.07 (5–76)	32.72 (4.5–76)	.5620

Abbreviations: EBL, estimated blood loss; LOS, length of stay.

these approaches for many years. Because the senior author does not use the posterior approach, a comparison involving that approach was not conducted.

Based on the results of this study and our encouraging experience with the DA approach over the past 8 years, the senior author uses the DA approach as the preferred method for primary elective THA. Any patient with end-stage arthritis, regardless of their body habitus, is a candidate for THA using the DA approach. However, there are some circumstances in which the DL approach is preferred to the DA approach. These circumstances include patients with hardware in the proximal femur (ie, dynamic hip screw) requiring removal through a lateral incision and deformity of the proximal femur in which an extended trochanteric osteotomy may be required. Although extended trochanteric osteotomy can be easily performed through the DA approach, the lack of double offset broach handles for most extensively coated femoral stems makes revision of femur through the DA approach challenging. Nevertheless, many revisions have been performed through this approach at our institution.

Patients undergoing THA using the DA approach become independent of the walking devices early. The faster recovery allows them to return to employment and driving earlier. The latter is not to be underestimated considering that many young and fully employed patients are increasingly undergoing THA.

In the current climate of health care with emphasis on cost reduction, it is conceivable that THA performed by trained surgeons may allow containment of some costs (ie, physical therapy) associated with the delivery of care following THA. The use of the DA approach, in which the muscles involved in ambulation are not disturbed, has allowed the need for physical therapy to be reduced following discharge from the hospital. At present more than two-thirds of our patients undergoing THA using the DA approach do not require any physical therapy

after discharge from the hospital. Any effort to minimize cost, enhance functional recovery, and allow quicker return to driving and work are all positives in the current health care system.

In an effort to minimize use of resources, the authors prefer to perform the DA approach THA using regular operating room tables. Besides saving money associated with the purchase of a specialized table, the use of a regular operating room table avoids the need for additional personnel to operate the specialized table.

This study involving a single surgeon at 1 institution using proper randomization allowed the set objectives to be accomplished. All patients in this study were subjected to the same preoperative and postoperative care protocols and none of the patients were preconditioned regarding the potential benefit of DA approach THA. Thus, every effort was made to minimize the influence of variables that could confound the findings and allow the importance of surgical approach in early functional recovery to be isolated. Although the possibility of a type II error (inadequate sample size) is always present in studies that fail to detect a difference in some of the reported outcomes, the authors think that inclusion of a large sample size in the current study may have averted such a statistical flaw. However, the effect size (20%) used for calculation of the sample size may have been too large. The effect size was determined based on the available literature and the authors did ensure that 25% more patients were included in each group to allow for possible attrition.

The authors think that the findings of the current prospective, randomized study are important for both the patients and the surgeons contemplating different surgical approaches to THA. It seems that the use of select surgical approaches may confer some benefits in early functional recovery but not in other measured parameters. These potential benefits need to be weighed against major problems that could occur with new surgical approaches to THA, particularly during the learning curve period.

REFERENCES

1. Lawlor M, Humphreys P, Morrow E, et al. Comparison of early postoperative functional levels following total hip replacement using minimally invasive versus standard incisions. A prospective randomized blinded trial. Clin Rehabil 2005;19(5): 465–74.
2. Bender B, Nogler M, Hozack WJ. Direct anterior approach for total hip arthroplasty. Orthop Clin North Am 2009;40(3):321–8.
3. Chimento GF, Pavone V, Sharrock N, et al. Minimally invasive total hip arthroplasty: a prospective randomized study. J Arthroplasty 2005;20:139–44.
4. Seng BE, Berend KR, Ajluni AF, et al. Anterior-supine minimally invasive total hip arthroplasty: defining the learning curve. Orthop Clin North Am 2009;40(3):343–50.
5. Greidanus NV, Chihab S, Garbuz DS, et al. Outcomes of minimally invasive anterolateral THA are not superior to those of minimally invasive direct lateral and posterolateral THA. Clin Orthop Relat Res 2013;471(2):463–71.
6. Restrepo C, Parvizi J, Pour AE, et al. Prospective randomized study of two surgical approaches for total hip arthroplasty. J Arthroplasty 2010;25(5): 671–9.e1.
7. Berend KR, Lombardi AV Jr, Seng BE, et al. Enhanced early outcomes with the anterior supine intermuscular approach in primary total hip arthroplasty. J Bone Joint Surg Am 2009;91(Suppl 6):107–20.
8. Meneghini RM, Smits SA. Early discharge and recovery with three minimally invasive total hip arthroplasty approaches: a preliminary study. Clin Orthop Relat Res 2009;467(6):1431–7.
9. Dobson F, Hinman RS, Roos EM, et al. OARSI recommended performance-based tests to assess physical function in people diagnosed with hip or knee osteoarthritis. Osteoarthritis Cartilage 2013; 21(8):1042–52.
10. Min B-W, Song K-S, Bae K-C, et al. The effect of stem alignment on results of total hip arthroplasty with a cementless tapered-wedge femoral component. J Arthroplasty 2008;23(3):418–23.
11. Barrett WP, Turner SE, Leopold JP. Prospective randomized study of direct anterior vs posterolateral approach for total hip arthroplasty. J Arthroplasty 2013;28(9):1634–8.
12. Nilsdotter AK, Lohmander LS, Klässbo M, et al. Hip disability and osteoarthritis outcome score (HOOS)–validity and responsiveness in total hip replacement. BMC Musculoskelet Disord 2003;4:10.
13. Mayr E, Nogler M, Benedetti M-G, et al. A prospective randomized assessment of earlier functional recovery in THA patients treated by minimally invasive direct anterior approach: a gait analysis study. Clin Biomech (Bristol, Avon) 2009;24(10): 812–8.
14. Nho SJ, Kymes SM, Callaghan JJ, et al. The burden of osteoarthritis in the United States: epidemiologic considerations. J Am Acad Orthop Surg 2013;21(Suppl 1):S1–6.
15. Hallert O, Li Y, Brismar H, et al. The direct anterior approach: initial experience of a minimally invasive technique for total hip arthroplasty. J Orthop Surg Res 2012;7:17.

Diagnosis of Periprosthetic Joint Infection Following Hip and Knee Arthroplasty

Javad Parvizi, MD, FRCS*, Safa Cyrus Fassihi, BS,
Mohammad A. Enayatollahi, MD

KEYWORDS

- Periprosthetic • Joint • Infection • Diagnosis • Definition • Algorithm • Serology • Aspiration

KEY POINTS

- In an effort to establish clear diagnostic criteria for periprosthetic joint infections, this article proposes a modification of the currently established American Academy of Orthopaedic Surgeons algorithm.
- A stepwise approach should be undertaken, starting with history, physical examination, radiography, erythrocyte sedimentation rate, and C-reactive protein level.
- If the diagnosis is still unclear, joint aspiration with analysis of synovial leukocyte count, polymorphonuclear cell percentage, leukocyte esterase levels, and pathogen cultures should be obtained.
- In the case of indolent infections, newer diagnostic modalities, such as alpha-defensin or interleukin-6, show great potential to complement current techniques in future clinical practice.

INTRODUCTION

Total hip arthroplasty (THA) is one of the most successful operations in the history of orthopedic surgery.[1] Modeled on the low-friction arthroplasty introduced by Sir John Charnley in 1961, the modern THA has relieved pain and improved quality of life for millions of individuals worldwide.[2]

Total knee arthroplasty (TKA) gained popularity shortly after the advent of the modern THA, and, in 1972, Insall[3] introduced the total condylar prosthesis, which laid the framework for the modern TKA. Despite these developments, knee replacements were less successful than their hip counterparts because of complications with prosthetic design, and it was not until the 1990s that the total knee replacement was considered a successful operation.[4]

Presently, THA and TKA are among the most effective and widely performed surgical operations, with close to 1 million THAs and TKAs performed in the United States annually.[5,6] The number of joint replacements performed each year is also growing rapidly, with a 174% and 673% increase in annual procedures projected by 2030 for THA and TKA, respectively.[6] Given the considerable growth and success of total joint replacements over the past several decades, there has been a major focus on minimizing surgical complications in order to further improve long-term outcomes and drive down costs.

Periprosthetic joint infection (PJI) remains a major cause of failure in THA and TKA, despite an incidence of less than 2% in most national centers.[7,8] For both THA and TKA, PJI is the third leading cause of primary failure,[9,10] the

Disclosure: The authors have no financial or commercial conflicts of interest to declare. No commercial entity paid or directed, or agreed to pay or direct, any benefits to any research fund, foundation, division, center, clinical practice, or other charitable or nonprofit organization with which the authors, or a member of their immediate families, are affiliated or associated.

Rothman Institute at Thomas Jefferson University Hospital, 925 Chestnut Street, Philadelphia, PA 19107, USA
* Corresponding author.
E-mail address: research@rothmaninstitute.com

0030-5898/16/$ – see front matter © 2016 Elsevier Inc. All rights reserved.

leading cause of revision failure,[11,12] and the leading cause of early primary failure (<5 years),[10,13] which is a pertinent issue because PJI-associated revision results in a mortality 5 times greater than in revision following aseptic failure.[14] Furthermore, the financial burden of PJI is significantly greater than in uninfected cases, with a 76% and 52% increase in cost for infected THA and TKA, respectively.[15] With the significant added strain on patient outcomes and health care costs, the accurate and timely diagnosis of PJI is critical to the progressive improvement of modern arthroplasty.

DIAGNOSTIC CRITERIA FOR PERIPROSTHETIC JOINT INFECTION

The diagnostic requirements for PJI have been a source of uncertainty in the past, with conflicting criteria resulting in the inability to form a universal clinical definition. In 2011, the Musculoskeletal Infection Society proposed a unique set of PJI criteria[16] that, following further revision, was accepted by the US Centers for Disease Control and Prevention.[17] Of note, because of discrepancies in the magnitude of clinically meaningful biomarker increases in acute (<6 weeks) versus chronic (>6 weeks) PJI, the International Consensus Meeting (ICM) on PJI suggested specific biomarker threshold values that are reflected in the minor criteria of PJI[18] in the definition given later.

DEFINITION OF PERIPROSTHETIC JOINT INFECTION

Joint or bursa infections must meet at least 1 of the following criteria:

1. Two positive periprosthetic (tissue or fluid) cultures with matching organisms.
2. A sinus tract communicating with the joint (Fig. 1).
3. Having 3 of the following minor criteria:
   a. Increased serum C-reactive protein (CRP) level (>100 mg/L in acute PJI; >10 mg/L in chronic PJI) and erythrocyte sedimentation rate (ESR; not applicable to acute PJI; >30 mm/h in chronic PJI)
   b. Increased synovial fluid white blood cell (WBC) count (>10,000 cells/μL in acute PJI; >3000 cells/μL in chronic PJI) or ++ (or greater) change on leukocyte esterase test strip of synovial fluid
   c. Increased synovial fluid polymorphonuclear neutrophil percentage (PMN%) (>90% in acute PJI; PMN% >80% in chronic PJI)

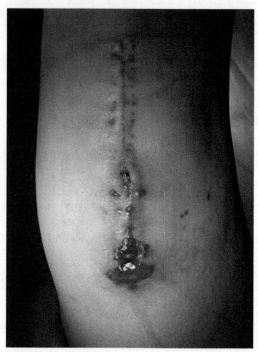

Fig. 1. Typical physical examination findings for PJI after TKA. Note the opening and drainage at the distal aspect of the incision.

   d. Positive histologic analysis of periprosthetic tissue (>5 neutrophils [PMNs] per high-power field [HPF])
   e. A single positive periprosthetic (tissue or fluid) culture

Even with the establishment of firm diagnostic criteria, the ICM noted that, if clinical suspicion for PJI is high, further diagnostic evaluation should commence even if the criteria listed earlier are not met in full.[18] For this reason, risk stratification, based on patient history, physical examination, and joint radiographs, is critical to establishing a diagnosis in cases lacking a straightforward diagnosis.

Also of note, The Society of Unicondylar Research and Continuing Education suggested that these criteria, including ESR and CRP threshold values, can also be used in suspected PJI following unicompartmental knee arthroplasty (UKA), but that the aspiration biomarker thresholds in UKA can deviate significantly from the ICM values for TKA.[19]

DIAGNOSTIC MODALITIES IN SUSPECTED PERIPROSTHETIC JOINT INFECTION

Before constructing a stepwise approach to diagnosing PJI, it is essential to understand the clinical utility of the various diagnostic modalities. The mainstays in the evaluation of PJI include:

1. Detailed history, physical examination, and risk factor identification
2. Joint radiographs
3. ESR and CRP serology
4. Joint aspiration and culture

Additional diagnostic tools are useful on a conditional basis and are discussed later.

AN ALGORITHMIC APPROACH TO DIAGNOSING PERIPROSTHETIC JOINT INFECTION

In order to apply the diagnostic modalities in an organized fashion while minimizing invasive interventions, the authors propose a modification of the American Academy of Orthopaedic Surgeons' diagnostic algorithm that accounts for more recent clinical data and recommendations[20,21] (Fig. 2). In all cases, this algorithm should not be used as a definitive diagnostic tool, but as an adjunct to clinical expertise and planned care. Furthermore, a high clinical suspicion should supersede any negative PJI diagnosis acquired through use of the algorithm.[18]

PATIENT HISTORY, PHYSICAL EXAMINATION, AND RISK FACTOR IDENTIFICATION

As with any postoperative complication, a focused history and physical is the first step in raising sufficient clinical suspicion for further work-up. For PJI, the clinical presentation varies significantly according to time frame and pathogen (Table 1).

Because of a lack of empirical evidence regarding risk stratification in suspected PJI,[21] underlying risk factors are another useful tool in stratifying patients into high-risk and low-risk categories.

Predisposing risk factors for periprosthetic joint infection[24–26]

- Local risk factors
  - Superficial surgical site infection
  - Joint malignancy
  - History of native joint septic arthritis
  - History of prior PJI
  - Prior arthroplasty of joint
  - Skin ulcers
  - Postoperative hematoma formation
- Systemic risk factors
  - National Nosocomial Infections Surveillance System surgical patient risk index score of 1 or 2

  - Systemic malignancy
  - Rheumatoid arthritis
  - Immunocompromised host
  - Diabetes mellitus
  - Increased body mass index
  - Intravenous drug use
  - Steroid therapy
  - Systemic skin conditions
  - Increased duration of surgery

IMAGING STUDIES

Owing to their ease of use, rapid turnover, low associated costs, and ability to rule out other causes of joint pain, plain radiographs are the imaging study of choice despite their low sensitivity and specificity in diagnosing PJI.[22,27] It is presently unclear whether or not computed tomography and MRI have a place in the routine diagnostic evaluation of PJI, because prosthesis-borne artifacts preclude reliable image interpretation, and the current MRI artifact reduction software is largely incapable of adequately ameliorating this issue.[21,22,28] The utility of ultrasonography is limited to PJI with significant local fluid accumulation,[29] and for PET scans and other forms of nuclear imaging further studies are needed, because the present data regarding accuracy are conflicting.[22,30,31] Leukocyte scans and bone scans are generally not recommended because of unavailability and invasiveness, respectively.[22,28]

Common radiographic findings in periprosthetic joint infection

- Focal osteolysis, as indicated by a widened (>2 mm) band of radiolucency at the metal-bone interface or cement-bone interface[22]
- Loosening of components, particularly in a rapid and aggressive fashion characteristic of infectious loosening (vs the slow progression of aseptic loosening)[32]
- Cement fractures[32]
- Subperiosteal reaction[32]

SERUM STUDIES: ERYTHROCYTE SEDIMENTATION RATE AND C-REACTIVE PROTEIN

It is the current recommendation that ESR and CRP be acquired in all cases of painful THA/TKA, because the combination of a normal ESR and CRP level is an excellent predictor of the absence of infection.[33] The sensitivity of a combined increase in both ESR and CRP level

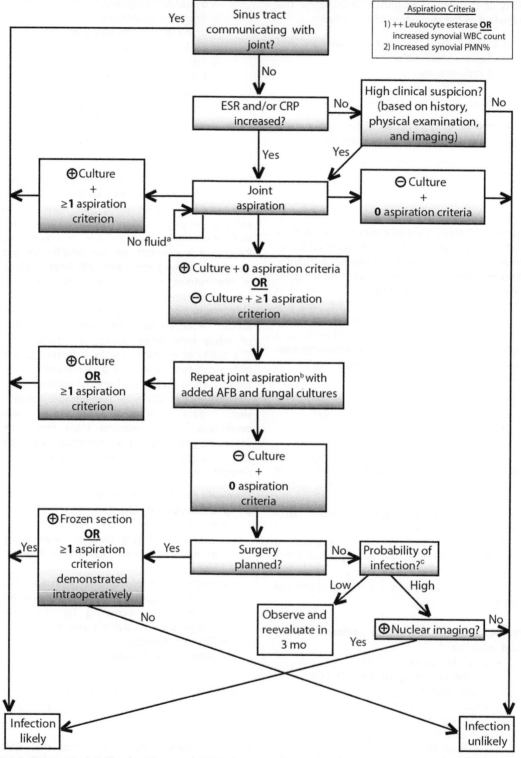

Fig. 2. Diagnostic algorithm for PJI. −, negative; +, positive; AFB, acid-fast bacilli. ªIf no fluid is drained, repeat aspiration. If 2 consecutive dry taps occur, proceed to biopsy with micro and histology. A + biopsy indicates likely infection and a − biopsy indicates unlikely infection. ᵇ Repeat joint aspiration is strongly encouraged in cases of high clinical suspicion, even in the absence of increased synovial biomarkers on initial aspiration. ᶜ As determined by history, physical examination, and radiography.

approaches 98% in detecting PJI.[34] However, ESR/CRP have numerous shortcomings:

1. Poor specificity,[35] because they are increased in numerous states of inflammation, from physiologic increases in the postoperative window to drawn-out cases with long-standing comorbidities
2. Clinical significance of ESR/CRP level increases are often confounded by patient demographics and laboratory testing methods[25]

In addition, recent research suggests that the combination of increased ESR and CRP level is not as robust in detecting PJI as was once thought, with a false-negative rate exceeding 11% in some cases.[35] This finding is further underscored by emerging evidence that infectious TKA failure is often misdiagnosed as being aseptic despite standard clinical work-up that includes ESR and CRP serology.[36] The divergent findings regarding the usefulness of ESR and CRP warrant further investigation and may be caused by the fact that:

1. Statistically optimized threshold values are paramount in establishing maximal sensitivity and specificity[37]
2. Low-virulence organisms (see Table 1; 3–12 month" latency post-THA/TKA) generate subtler increases in inflammatory biomarkers[25]

Table 1
Common findings in history, physical examination, culture, and mode of pathogenic entry as determined by time after arthroplasty

Time After Surgery (mo)	History	Physical Examination	Culture	Likely Mode of Entry
<3	*Rapid* onset of joint pain and/or stiffness	1. Cardinal signs of infection (edema, erythema, warmth, tenderness, and/or fever) are often present 2. Effusion, wound dehiscence, or site drainage may be noted 3. Superficial necrosis, cellulitis, and hematoma formation often accompany acute PJI[22]	High-virulence pathogens; ie, *Staphylococcus aureus* or gram-negative bacilli	Operative implantation or postoperative wound dehiscence
3–12	*Slow, progressive* joint pain and/or stiffness	1. Often clinically indistinguishable from aseptic prosthesis failure 2. A sinus tract communicating with the joint may be observed	Low-virulence pathogens; ie, *Propionibacterium acnes* or coagulase-negative *Staphylococcus*	Operative implantation
>12	1. *Rapid* onset of joint pain and stiffness 2. Patient may recall a distant site of infection/trauma or history of bacteremia (roughly half of all cases[23]) 3. Joint was previously more functional and less painful	Cardinal signs of infection (edema, erythema, warmth, tenderness, and/or fever) may be present	*S aureus*, *Streptococcus* spp, or gram-negative bacilli[23]	Hematogenous seeding

3. ESR has no diagnostic utility in acute PJI (<6 weeks)[18]

DIAGNOSTIC ARTHROCENTESIS WITH SYNOVIAL BIOMARKERS

If the initial battery of screening tests (history, physical examination, imaging, and inflammatory biomarkers) are suggestive of PJI, the next step is a joint aspiration with analysis of synovial WBC count, PMN%, leukocyte esterase levels, and synovial fluid cultures.[28] The joint aspiration may require radiographic guidance in THA and in cases of TKA with patients who are morbidly obese or have excessive scar tissue at the site.[38] Physicians should observe proper sterile technique, because species in the natural skin flora, like *Staphylococcus aureus*, are a major cause of PJI, and introduction of epidermal *S aureus* into the joint could not only yield false-positive culture results but could also result in iatrogenic PJI.[38]

Synovial WBC count and PMN% are highly accurate testing modalities, with lower WBC counts (1100/μL) having higher sensitivity and lower specificity (91% and 88%, respectively), and higher WBC counts (4200/μL) having lower sensitivity and higher specificity (84% and 93%, respectively).[39–42] Furthermore, a PMN% greater than 65% retains high sensitivity (97%) and specificity (98%) for PJI.[41] Much like ESR/CRP, synovial WBC count and PMN% increase after surgery universally, and thus adherence to threshold values with sufficient clinical data is prudent[18,43] (discussed earlier); however, there is no variation in these threshold values in patients with chronic inflammatory disorders.[44]

In order to attain an accurate leukocyte count, a formula was devised by Ghanem and colleagues[45] to identify the true leukocyte count (adjusted WBC), with *blood* denoting blood values, *fluid* denoting synovial fluid values, *observed WBC* denoting the number of WBC present in the synovial fluid, and *expected WBC* denoting the number of WBC theoretically introduced into the joint via traumatic tap:

$$\text{Expected WBC} = (\text{WBC}_{blood}/\text{RBC}_{blood}) \times \text{RBC}_{fluid}$$

$$\text{Adjusted WBC} = \text{observed WBC} - \text{expected WBC}$$

In addition, the WBC differential may be influenced by free metal debris, as seen in failed metal-on-metal bearings or in cases of corrosion.[25] In such scenarios, the monocytes phagocytosing the metallic debris get falsely identified as neutrophils by the automated machinery,[46] necessitating a manual WBC count to rectify the falsely increased PMN count.[18]

LEUKOCYTE ESTERASE

As in the urine dipstick test, leukocyte esterase (LE) is an enzyme released by neutrophils in response to an infection. According to preliminary data, it remains an accurate test for infection at numerous sites, and with regard to PJI, an LE of ++ has a:

- Sensitivity of 81%
- Specificity of 100%
- Positive predictive value of 100%
- Negative predictive value of 93%
- Strong correlation with ESR, CRP, synovial WBC count, and synovial PMN%[47]

The test is rapid and inexpensive, and it involves simply immersing a urine test strip in synovial fluid and reading the color change after 2 minutes (Fig. 3).

In cases of bloody joint aspirations, 1.5 mL of synovial fluid should be transferred to a microcentrifuge tube, loaded into a minicentrifuge symmetrically, and spun for 2 to 3 minutes at maximum speed (ideally ≥6600 revolutions per minute). The synovial fluid separates as the supernatant, which can be needle aspirated and transferred for accurate LE testing.[48]

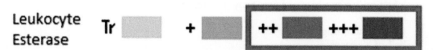

Fig. 3. The Leukocyte Esterase (LE) test - Under the "Leukocytes" row of a urinary dipstick, a "++" or higher color change indicates a positive result (represented by the red box). Anything less than a "++" is considered a negative result with this testing method.

SYNOVIAL FLUID CULTURE

As part of the synovial fluid analysis, cultures should be obtained in order to properly direct therapy to the infecting microorganism. The test is accurate, with the sensitivity of synovial fluid culture ranging from 86% to 92% and the specificity ranging from 82% to 97%.[40,49,50]

At least 3 samples should be obtained and sent for aerobic/anaerobic culture, with culture of synovial fluid in blood culture vials (sensitivity 90%–92%) being preferred to intraoperative swab cultures (sensitivity 68%–76%) and tissue cultures (sensitivity 77%–82%).[51] Additional mycobacterial and fungal cultures can be obtained for at-risk patients or when clinical suspicion dictates such action[52,53] but, at present, these cultures are not even useful in cases of culture-negative PJI.[54] In cases of cultures that yield low-virulence organisms, a repeat culture is recommended to rule out contamination.[52]

For optimal culture results, antibiotics should be held for at least 2 weeks before obtaining the cultures,[55] and although routine 5-day cultures are sufficient for many patients, extending cultures to at least 2 weeks has been shown to improve yields in culture-negative PJI.[51,56] Importantly, antibiotics should still be administered preoperatively even if obtaining cultures, because the sensitivity of intraoperative cultures is unaffected by antimicrobial prophylaxis.[57] The only cases in which preoperative antibiotics should be withheld are in culture-negative PJI for which clinical suspicion remains high.[18]

HISTOPATHOLOGY: A MINOR CRITERION FOR DIAGNOSING PERIPROSTHETIC JOINT INFECTION

In performing a histopathologic analysis, samples should be obtained using sharp dissection rather than cautery to limit false-positive results.[18,25] An acute inflammatory reaction, more accurately defined as 5 to 10 PMN per HPF in at least 5 HPF, is an accurate predictor of culture-positive PJI (likelihood ratio [LR] of 12.0).[58] In contrast, histology has an LR of only 0.23 in diagnosing culture-negative PJI[58] and thus should be used with caution in such cases. Of note, a combined total of 23 PMN in 10 HPF is the diagnostic equivalent of 5 to 10 PMN per HPF in at least 5 HPF.[59]

TISSUE BIOPSY AND CULTURE

In cases of negative synovial fluid cultures with high remaining clinical suspicion, tissue sampling with cultures may be obtained. The ICM recommends acquiring 3 to 5 samples of tissue or fluid,[52] with acceptable forms of tissue acquisition including preoperative or intraoperative tissue removal, including both open and arthroscopic approaches. Biopsy is always preferred to swab cultures, because the latter have low sensitivity.[52,60]

PROSPECTIVE DIAGNOSTIC MODALITIES: THE FUTURE OF DIAGNOSING PERIPROSTHETIC JOINT INFECTION

There are numerous emerging advancements that may replace or supplement the established diagnostic tools in imaging, laboratory markers, and cultures.

Imaging

At present, PET scans are significant only in the research realm of diagnosing PJI, owing in part to the conflicting data regarding the accuracy of PET scan.[22,30,31] With many studies reporting highly divergent values for PET scan accuracy, additional trials are needed to validate the role of the PET scan in the routine diagnostic workup of PJI. This stance regarding the requirement of further study was reaffirmed in 2008, when a meta-analysis of 11 studies concluded that although the pooled sensitivity and specificity of fluorodeoxyglucose-PET in infected THA/TKA was 82.1% and 86.6%, respectively, there was an unusual amount of heterogeneity among the reported results of the analyzed studies.[61] Nonetheless, the potential of PET scans is of major interest, because recent trials, such as that conducted by Kobayashi and colleagues,[62] have shown a sensitivity of 95% and a specificity of 98% in diagnosing PJI.

Serologic Biomarkers

Although ESR/CRP are still standard of care concerning laboratory values in the screening of PJI, a recent meta-analysis on inflammatory markers in PJI suggested that interleukin-6 (IL-6) is stronger than ESR/CRP in aiding clinicians in the diagnosis of PJI, because increased postsurgical IL-6 levels return to baseline in a matter of days.[63] Specifically, the diagnostic odds ratio of IL-6 was 314.7, compared with only 13.1 and 7.2 for CRP and ESR, respectively.[63] However, further trials are required before IL-6 should be considered a component of routine PJI workup, because the meta-analysis was limited by the number of studies on IL-6 (3) versus the number of studies on CRP (23) and ESR (25).

Joint Aspirate Biomarkers

Regarding the inflammatory marker CRP, Parvizi and colleagues[64] recently showed that an enzyme-linked immunosorbent assay (ELISA) of synovial CRP test dramatically improves the diagnostic accuracy relative to the traditional serum CRP assay. The sensitivity and specificity of the synovial multiplex assay was 85% and 97% versus 76% and 93% for the serum assay.[64] Typically, by the time joint aspiration takes place, a CRP test has already been drawn from the serum, but in cases in which infection is suspected but serum CRP level is subthreshold, an additional synovial CRP test via ELISA assay could potentially solidify a PJI diagnosis.

Alpha-defensin, a peptide secreted by human cells in response to microbial products, is another marker that can be detected in the synovial fluid. Unlike the traditional inflammatory biomarkers, alpha-defensin levels are not influenced by systemic inflammation, and although antibiotic therapy can preclude diagnosis via joint/tissue culture, alpha-defensin levels remain unaffected by antimicrobial therapy.[25,65,66] For this reason, the alpha-defensin immunoassay remains a promising laboratory technique, and, when using the established threshold value of 5.2 mg/L,[65] the test has shown a sensitivity and specificity of 100%.[25,65,66]

Culture of Pathogens

The culture of a pathogen from joint or tissue aspirates remains an imperfect diagnostic tool, owing to several confounding factors, including prior antibiotic therapy, low inoculum, fastidious microorganisms, and the formation of biofilms.

One solution to the issues surrounding both biofilms and perioperative antibiotics is sonication of the explanted prosthesis, which effectively dislodges bacteria from the prosthesis biofilm for easier access. In a 2007 prospective trial comparing sonicate-fluid cultures with traditional cultures, sonicate-fluid cultures had equivalent specificity (99%) and improved sensitivity (79% vs 61%).[67] The improvement in sensitivity was even greater in those patients who received antimicrobial therapy within 14 days before surgery (75% vs 45%).[67] Explant sonication seems to provide a remarkable improvement compared with traditional culturing techniques, but the technique is not routine in most laboratories at present.

One means of identifying a pathogen in PJI without culture is through polymerase chain reaction (PCR).[68–71] The PCR is typically either specific only for a single microorganism or broad range (16S ribosomal DNA) for unknown organisms, and although the broad-range PCR seems to be mechanistically suitable for identifying a pathogen in PJI, it is limited by a high incidence of false-positive results, inability to detect polymicrobial infection, and the added strain of subsequent sequencing for pathogen identification.[72] These issues are largely ameliorated by the advent of the Ibis T500 Universal Biosensor, which combines broad-range PCR with high-performance electrospray ionization mass spectrometry. In doing so, the Ibis T5000 outperforms conventional PCR and has the ability to detect bacteria, viruses, fungi, and protozoa[73]; however, it retains the high false-positive rate of conventional PCR.[36] The biosensor is not approved by the US Food and Drug Administration at present, but it holds promise in diagnosing culture-negative suspected PJI in the future.[36]

SUMMARY

With a new gold-standard definition of PJI and an evidence-based diagnostic algorithm to guide diagnosis, the proper evaluation and subsequent treatment of PJI stands to improve even further in the near future. Despite this progress, a concrete diagnosis of PJI remains elusive, and clinical acumen should outweigh diagnostic tests when suspicion for infection is high. As the body of research catches up to the available prospective diagnostic technologies, diagnosing PJI in complex cases may become clearer and more accurate in the coming years.

REFERENCES

1. Callaghan JJ, Albright JC, Goetz DD, et al. Charnley total hip arthroplasty with cement. Minimum twenty-five-year follow-up. J Bone Joint Surg Am 2000;82(4):487–97.

2. Knight SR, Aujla R, Biswas SP. Total hip arthroplasty – over 100 years of operative history. Orthop Rev (Pavia) 2011;3(2):E16.

3. Insall JN, Clarke HD. Historical development, classification, and characteristics of knee prostheses. In: Insall JN, Clarke HD, editors. Insall & Scott Surgery of the Knee. 3rd edition. New York: Churchill Livingstone; 2001. p. 1516–52.

4. Moran CG, Horton TC. Total knee replacement: the joint of the decade. BMJ 2000;320(7238):820. Web.

5. Pivec R, Johnson AJ, Mears SC, et al. Hip arthroplasty. Lancet 2012;380(9855):1768–77.

6. Kurtz S, Ong K, Lau E, et al. Projections of primary and revision hip and knee arthroplasty in the United States from 2005 to 2030. J Bone Joint Surg Am 2007;89(4):780–5.

7. Namba RS, Inacio MC, Paxton EW. Risk factors associated with deep surgical site infections after primary total knee arthroplasty. J Bone Joint Surg Am 2013;95(9):775–82.

8. NIH consensus conference: total hip replacement. NIH consensus development panel on total hip replacement. JAMA 1995;273(24):1950–6.

9. Ulrich SD, Seyler TM, Bennett D, et al. Total hip arthroplasties: what are the reasons for revision? Int Orthop 2007;32(5):597–604.

10. Narkbunnam R, Chareancholvanich K. Causes of failure in total knee arthroplasty. J Med Assoc Thai 2012;95(5):667–73.

11. Jafari SM, Coyle C, Mortazavi SM, et al. Revision hip arthroplasty: infection is the most common cause of failure. Clin Orthop Relat Res 2010; 468(8):2046–51.

12. Mortazavi SM, Molligan J, Austin MS, et al. Failure following revision total knee arthroplasty: infection is the major cause. Int Orthop 2010;35(8):1157–64.

13. Iamthanaporn K, Chareancholvanich K, Pornrattanamaneewong C. Revision primary total hip replacement: causes and risk factors. J Med Assoc Thai 2015;98(1):93–9.

14. Zmistowski B, Karam JA, Durinka JB, et al. Periprosthetic joint infection increases the risk of one-year mortality. J Bone Joint Surg Am 2013; 95(24):2177–84.

15. Kurtz SM, Lau E, Schmier J, et al. Infection burden for hip and knee arthroplasty in the United States. J Arthroplasty 2008;23(7):984–91.

16. Parvizi J, Zmistowski B, Berbari EF, et al. New definition for periprosthetic joint infection: from the workgroup of the Musculoskeletal Infection Society. Clin Orthop Relat Res 2011;469(11):2992–4.

17. CDC - ACH Surveillance for surgical site infection (SSI) event – NHSN. Available at: http://www.cdc.gov/nhsn/PDFs/pscManual/17pscNosInfDef_current.pdf. Accessed August 3, 2015.

18. Zmistowski B, Della Valle C, Bauer TW, et al. Diagnosis of periprosthetic joint infection. J Arthroplasty 2014; 29(Suppl 2):77–83.

19. Society of Unicondylar Research and Continuing Education. Diagnosis of periprosthetic joint infection after unicompartmental knee arthroplasty. J Arthroplasty 2012;27(8):46–50.

20. Diaz-Ledezma C, Lichstein PM, Dolan JG, et al. Diagnosis of periprosthetic joint infection in Medicare patients: multicriteria decision analysis. Clin Orthop Relat Res 2014;472(11):3275–84.

21. Della Valle C, Parvizi J, Bauer TW, et al, American Academy of Orthopaedic Surgeons. Diagnosis of periprosthetic joint infections of the hip and knee. J Am Acad Orthop Surg 2010;18(12):760–70.

22. Lima AL, Oliveira PR, Carvalho VC, et al. Periprosthetic joint infections. Interdiscip Perspect Infect Dis 2013;2013:542796.

23. Rodríguez D, Pigrau C, Euba G, et al. Acute haematogenous prosthetic joint infection: prospective evaluation of medical and surgical management. Clin Microbiol Infect 2010;16(12):1789–95.

24. Berbari EF, Hanssen AD, Duffy MC, et al. Risk factors for prosthetic joint infection: case-control study. Clin Infect Dis 1998;27(5):1247–54.

25. Enayatollahi MA, Parvizi J. Diagnosis of infected total hip arthroplasty. Hip Int 2015;25(4):294–300.

26. Poss R, Thornhill TS, Ewald FC, et al. Factors influencing the incidence and outcome of infection following total joint arthroplasty. Clin Orthop Relat Res 1984;(182):117–26.

27. Osmon DR, Berbari EF, Berendt AR, et al. Diagnosis and management of prosthetic joint infection: clinical practice guidelines by the Infectious Diseases Society of America. Clin Infect Dis 2013;56:e1–25.

28. Osmon DR, Berbari EF, Berendt AR, et al. Executive summary: diagnosis and management of prosthetic joint infection: clinical practice guidelines by the Infectious Diseases Society of America. Clin Infect Dis 2012;56(1):1–10.

29. Sofka CM. Current applications of advanced cross-sectional imaging techniques in evaluating the painful arthroplasty. Skeletal Radiol 2007;36(3): 183–93.

30. Chryssikos T, Parvizi J, Ghanem E, et al. FDG-PET imaging can diagnose periprosthetic infection of the hip. Clin Orthop Relat Res 2008;466(6):1338–42.

31. Sousa R, Massada M, Pereira A, et al. Diagnostic accuracy of combined 99mTc-sulesomab and 99mTc-nanocolloid bone marrow imaging in detecting prosthetic joint infection. Nucl Med Commun 2011;32(9):834–9.

32. Tigges S, Stiles RG, Roberson JR. Appearance of septic hip prostheses on plain radiographs. AJR Am J Roentgenol 1994;163(2):377–80.

33. Spangehl MJ, Masri BA, O'Connell JX, et al. Prospective analysis of preoperative and intraoperative investigations for the diagnosis of infection at the sites of two hundred and two revision total hip arthroplasties. J Bone Joint Surg Am 1999; 81(5):672.

34. Ghanem E, Antoci V, Pulido L, et al. The use of receiver operating characteristics analysis in determining erythrocyte sedimentation rate and c-reactive protein levels in diagnosing periprosthetic infection prior to revision total hip arthroplasty. Int J Infect Dis 2009;13(6):e444–9.

35. Johnson AJ, Zywiel MG, Stroh A, et al. Serological markers can lead to false negative diagnoses of periprosthetic infections following total knee arthroplasty. Int Orthop 2010;35(11):1621–6.

36. Rasouli MR, Harandi AA, Adeli B, et al. Revision total knee arthroplasty: infection should be ruled out in all cases. J Arthroplasty 2012;27(6):1239–43.e1-2.

37. Greidanus NV, Masri BA, Garbuz DS, et al. Use of erythrocyte sedimentation rate and C-reactive protein level to diagnose infection before revision total knee arthroplasty. A prospective evaluation. J Bone Joint Surg Am 2007;89:1409.

38. Squire MW, Della Valle CJ, Parvizi J, et al. Preoperative diagnosis of periprosthetic joint infection: role of aspiration. AJR Am J Roentgenol 2011;196(4): 875–9.

39. Bedair H, Ting N, Jacovides C, et al. The Mark Coventry Award: diagnosis of early postoperative TKA infection using synovial fluid analysis. Clin Orthop Relat Res 2011;469(1):34–40.

40. Schinsky MF, Della Valle CJ, Sporer SM, et al. Perioperative testing for joint infection in patients undergoing revision total hip arthroplasty. J Bone Joint Surg Am 2008;90(9):1869–75.

41. Trampuz A, Hanssen AD, Osmon DR, et al. Synovial fluid leukocyte count and differential for the diagnosis of prosthetic knee infection. Am J Med 2004;117(8):556–62.

42. Ghanem E, Parvizi J, Burnett RS, et al. Cell count and differential of aspirated fluid in the diagnosis of infection at the site of total knee arthroplasty. J Bone Joint Surg Am 2008;90(8):1637.

43. Parvizi J, Jacovides C, Zmistowski B, et al. Definition of periprosthetic joint infection: is there a consensus? Clin Orthop Relat Res 2011;469(11):3022–30.

44. Cipriano CA, Brown NM, Michael AM, et al. Serum and synovial fluid analysis for diagnosing chronic periprosthetic infection in patients with inflammatory arthritis. J Bone Joint Surg Am 2012;94(7):594–600.

45. Ghanem E, Houssock C, Pulido L, et al. Determining "true" leukocytosis in bloody joint aspiration. J Arthroplasty 2008;23(2):182–7.

46. Wyles CC, Larson DR, Houdek MT, et al. Utility of synovial fluid aspirations in failed metal-on-metal total hip arthroplasty. J Arthroplasty 2013;28(5):818–23.

47. Parvizi J, Jacovides C, Antoci V, et al. Diagnosis of periprosthetic joint infection: the utility of a simple yet unappreciated enzyme. J Bone Joint Surg Am 2011;93(24):2242–8.

48. Aggarwal VK, Tischler E, Ghanem E, et al. Leukocyte esterase from synovial fluid aspirate: a technical note. J Arthroplasty 2013;28(1):193–5.

49. Lachiewicz PF, Rogers GD, Thomason HC. Aspiration of the hip joint before revision total hip arthroplasty. clinical and laboratory factors influencing attainment of a positive culture. J Bone Joint Surg Am 1996;78(5):749.

50. Spangehl MJ, Younger AS, Masri BA, et al. Diagnosis of infection following total hip arthroplasty. Instr Course Lect 1998;47:285–95.

51. Larsen LH, Lange J, Xu Y, et al. Optimizing culture methods for diagnosis of prosthetic joint infections: a summary of modifications and improvements reported since 1995. J Med Microbiol 2012;61(3): 309–16.

52. Atkins BL, Athanasou N, Deeks JJ, et al. Prospective evaluation of criteria for microbiological diagnosis of prosthetic-joint infection at revision arthroplasty. J Clin Microbiol 1998;36(10):2932.

53. Wadey VM, Huddleston JI, Goodman SB, et al. Use and cost-effectiveness of intraoperative acid-fast bacilli and fungal cultures in assessing infection of joint arthroplasties. J Arthroplasty 2010;25(8): 1231–4.

54. Tokarski AT, O'Neil J, Deirmengian CA, et al. The routine use of atypical cultures in presumed aseptic revisions is unnecessary. Clin Orthop Relat Res 2013;471(10):3171–7.

55. Malekzadeh D, Osmon DR, Lahr BD, et al. Prior use of antimicrobial therapy is a risk factor for culture-negative prosthetic joint infection. Clin Orthop Relat Res 2010;468(8):2039–45.

56. Schwotzer N, Wahl P, Fracheboud D, et al. Optimal culture incubation time in orthopedic device-associated infections: a retrospective analysis of prolonged 14-day incubation. J Clin Microbiol 2014;52(1):61–6.

57. Ghanem E, Parvizi J, Clohisy J, et al. Perioperative antibiotics should not be withheld in proven cases of periprosthetic infection. Clin Orthop Relat Res 2007;461(461):44–7.

58. Tsaras G, Maduka-Ezeh A, Inwards CY, et al. Utility of Intraoperative frozen section histopathology in the diagnosis of periprosthetic joint infection. J Bone Joint Surg Am 2012;94(18):1700–11.

59. Morawietz L, Tiddens O, Mueller M, et al. Twenty-three neutrophil granulocytes in 10 high-power fields is the best histopathological threshold to differentiate between aseptic and septic endoprosthesis loosening. Histopathology 2009;54(7):847–53.

60. Zimmerli W, Trampuz A, Ochsner PE. Prosthetic-joint Infections. N Engl J Med 2004;351(16):1645.

61. Kwee TC, Kwee RM, Alavi A. FDG-PET for diagnosing prosthetic joint infection: systematic review and metaanalysis. Eur J Nucl Med Mol Imaging 2008;35(11):2122–32.

62. Kobayashi N, Inaba Y, Choe H, et al. Use of F-18 fluoride PET to differentiate septic from aseptic loosening in total hip arthroplasty patients. Clin Nucl Med 2011;36(11):e156–61.

63. Berbari E, Mabry T, Tsaras G, et al. Inflammatory blood laboratory levels as markers of prosthetic joint infection: a systematic review and meta-analysis. J Bone Joint Surg Am 2010;92(11):2102–9.

64. Parvizi J, Jacovides C, Adeli B, et al. Coventry Award: synovial C-reactive protein: a prospective evaluation of a molecular marker for periprosthetic knee joint infection. Clin Orthop Relat Res 2012; 470(1):54–60.

65. Deirmengian C, Kardos K, Kilmartin P, et al. The alpha-defensin test for periprosthetic joint infection outperforms the leukocyte esterase test strip. Clin Orthop Relat Res 2015;473(1):198–203.

66. Deirmengian C, Kardos K, Kilmartin P, et al. Diagnosing periprosthetic joint infection: has the era

of the biomarker arrived? Clin Orthop Relat Res 2014;472(11):3254–62.

67. Trampuz A, Piper KE, Jacobson MJ, et al. Sonication of removed hip and knee prostheses for diagnosis of infection. N Engl J Med 2007; 357(7):654–63.

68. Tunney MM, Patrick S, Curran MD, et al. Detection of prosthetic 287 hip infection at revision arthroplasty by immunofluorescence microscopy and PCR amplification of the bacterial 16S rRNA gene. J Clin Microbiol 1999;37:3281.

69. Panousis K, Grigoris P, Butcher I, et al. Poor predictive value of broad-range PCR for the detection of arthroplasty infection in 92 cases. Acta Orthop 2005;76:341.

70. Levine MJ, Mariani BA, Tuan RS, et al. Molecular genetic diagnosis of infected total joint arthroplasty. J Arthroplasty 1995;10:93.

71. Mariani BD, Martin DS, Levine MJ, et al. The Coventry Award. Polymerase chain reaction detection of bacterial infection in total knee arthroplasty. Clin Orthop Relat Res 1996;(331):11.

72. Achermann Y, Vogt M, Leunig M, et al. Improved diagnosis of periprosthetic joint infection by multiplex PCR of sonication fluid from removed implants. J Clin Microbiol 2010;48(4): 1208–14.

73. Ecker DJ, Sampath R, Massire C, et al. Ibis T5000: a universal biosensor approach for microbiology. Nat Rev Microbiol 2008;6(7):553–8.

Trauma

Acute Compartment Syndrome

Andrew H. Schmidt, MD

KEYWORDS

- Acute compartment syndrome • Fasciotomy • Intramuscular pressure • Perfusion pressure
- Pressure monitoring • Complication

KEY POINTS

- Frequent clinical assessment of patients considered to be at risk for developing compartment syndrome, ideally using a structured checklist, remains the cornerstone of diagnosis. In alert patients, monitoring of limb swelling, pain (both at rest and with passive muscle stretching), and neurologic status provides clues to the onset of acute compartment syndrome (ACS). The clinical findings are of greatest utility when several findings are present together.
- When a patient is unconscious or otherwise not able to be clinically assessed at frequent intervals, then continuous measurement of intramuscular pressure within the anterior compartment is of benefit. Continuous pressure monitoring, using a threshold for fasciotomy of a perfusion pressure (diastolic pressure minus muscle pressure) sustained at less than 30 mm Hg for 2 hours, has a 93% positive predictive value for the diagnosis of ACS.
- Although based primarily on retrospective studies, the literature is convincing that, when compartment syndrome is going to occur, early fasciotomy can avoid myonecrosis or ischemic neuropathy. However, the challenges in diagnosis, and the fact that compartment syndrome does not begin at a well-defined point in time, make it impossible to draw specific conclusions about the optimum timing of fasciotomy.

INTRODUCTION

Nature of the Problem

Acute compartment syndrome (ACS) is a complication of trauma or tissue ischemia, and can potentially involve any myofascial compartment in the body, whether in the extremities or trunk. Compartment syndrome most often occurs following a fracture or a crush injury to the limb.[1] When muscle swelling occurs following such injury, or with muscle reperfusion following a period of ischemia, the mass within the myofascial compartment increases because of accumulation of blood and other tissue fluids. Because of the inelastic nature of muscle fascia and other connective tissues, this accumulation of mass leads to increased pressure within the compartment, which is transmitted to the thin-walled venous system, causing venous hypertension and further transudation of fluid.[2] Progressive tissue ischemia and necrosis ensues, with eventual irreversible ischemic injury to all of the myoneural tissues within the involved compartment.

Despite ACS being well known and most clinicians being aware of its potential limb-threatening nature, it is a progressive phenomenon, and there is no standard definition of when compartment begins. The standard clinical signs and symptoms of ACS are pain and swelling, which are just as common in patients without ACS.[3] It is possible to quantify intramuscular pressure by direct measurement,[4,5] but both the clinical findings of ACS and measurement of intramuscular pressure have significant pitfalls as a means of diagnosis.[3,6–13] As a result, there is

Disclosure: The author received no funds in support of this article. The author has received research funding from the Dept. of Defense (W81XWH-10-1-0750, W81XWH-10-2-0090, W81XWH-12-1-0212). The author owns stock in Twin Star ECS.

Department of Orthopaedic Surgery, Hennepin County Medical Center, 701 Park Avenue South, Mail Code G2, Minneapolis, MN 55415, USA

E-mail address: schmi115@umn.edu

significant variation in the diagnosis of ACS and the frequency with which fasciotomy is performed.[14,15] Compartment syndrome is one of the most common causes of litigation against orthopedic surgeons.[16]

The only effective treatment of ACS is immediate decompressive surgical fasciotomy, wherein the skin and muscle fascia of the involved compartment are incised the length of the compartment in order to release the constricting soft tissues and increase the volume of the muscle compartment, thereby causing immediate reduction of compartment pressure and restoring perfusion. It has been estimated that muscle necrosis may occur within 2 hours of injury in as many as 35% of patients with ACS.[17] It is widely considered that performing early fasciotomy is critical to achieving the best possible outcomes when compartment syndrome occurs,[18–23] and it is generally accepted that performing unnecessary fasciotomy is better than missing a true case of compartment syndrome.

INDICATIONS/CONTRAINDICATIONS FOR EMERGENCY FASCIOTOMY

The only effective treatment of ACS is immediate fasciotomy, but if fasciotomy is performed the patient is committed to further surgery, a prolonged hospital stay, increased cost of care,[24,25] and increased morbidity.[21] Thus, clinicians facing patients at risk of ACS must choose a treatment plan from among several bad choices: perform fasciotomy and expose the patient to the risks and costs associated with that procedure, or not do fasciotomy and expose the patient to the potential adverse effects of delayed fasciotomy or missed ACS. Because of the latter, the primary indication for fasciotomy is a reasonable clinical assessment that the patient's examination is deteriorating, or that the patient is at risk of ACS and cannot be reliable followed from a clinical perspective.

Given that the diagnostic stakes are high and that there is some uncertainty in the diagnosis of ACS, understanding the risk factors for compartment syndrome allows surgeons to raise or lower the threshold for fasciotomy in a given clinical scenario. Young men sustaining high-energy trauma, especially of the lower leg and forearm, are considered to be the most at risk for compartment syndrome,[1] and a recent analysis suggests that young age is the strongest predictor.[26] ACS can occur without fracture, and such patients are older and have more medical comorbidities than those with a fracture.[19] Fracture pattern and location are also important.

Park and colleagues[27] evaluated 414 acute tibial fractures and compared rate of ACS requiring fasciotomy according to fracture location. ACS was most common in mid-diaphyseal tibia fractures (8% of cases), compared with proximal and distal metaphyseal fractures (<2% each).[27] Several series report an appreciable incidence of compartment syndrome in patients with tibial plateau fractures,[28] and these fractures must also be considered in the high-risk category. In addition, ACS occurs in slightly more than half (53%) of patients with medial knee fracture-dislocations and 18% of patients with bicondylar tibial plateau fractures treated with knee-spanning external fixation.[29]

The indication for fasciotomy is the diagnosis of early or impending ACS, but ACS is an entity without a definitive diagnostic test. The clinical diagnosis of ACS is best made using specific clinical findings (Box 1). However, the published literature makes it clear that these clinical signs and symptoms are unreliable, whether they are present[3,30] or absent.[31,32]

Given the lack of diagnostic certainty assigned to clinical signs and symptoms,[3] it makes sense to use objective evidence to diagnose ACS and decide when fasciotomy is needed. Compartment pressure monitoring has been advocated since the 1970s,[4,33] but the literature has not been able to provide consensus recommendations on what pressure thresholds were best used for fasciotomy.[10] The use of a pressure threshold for fasciotomy that is based on muscle perfusion pressure rather than on an absolute value of muscle pressure is more relevant physiologically and more specific.[34] The perfusion pressure (also referred to as the delta P) is defined as the difference between the patient's diastolic blood pressure and the intracompartment pressure.

Box 1
Specific clinical signs and symptoms used to diagnose ACS

- Tenseness or firmness of the involved compartment.
- Motor weakness.
- Pain with passive stretch of the involved muscle.
- Increasing pain and pain that is out-of-proportion to that expected.
- Loss of sensation in a specific neuronal distribution for a given compartment (eg, the deep peroneal nerve for the anterior compartment of the leg).

Fasciotomy may be safely avoided as long as the perfusion pressure remains greater than 30 mm Hg.[34] Typically, the anterior compartment is monitored because the pressures within it are typically highest.[35]

In the past, measurement of muscle pressure has been considered most valuable in patients who cannot be evaluated clinically, or have equivocal findings. Single pressure measurements alone are not representative of temporal changes in muscle pressure, and serial or continuous measurements showing increasing muscle pressure or decreasing perfusion pressure are likely to be more specific for patients who have compartment syndrome. Routine continuous pressure monitoring has been shown to dramatically reduce the rate of fasciotomy while avoiding cases with evidence of missed ACS.[34] Janzing and Broos[8] warned that routine use of continuous compartment pressure monitoring may increase the rate of fasciotomy,[8,36] and the literature suggests that the overall rate of fasciotomy is higher when continuous pressure monitoring is used compared with other methods.[37]

McQueen and colleagues,[34] in Edinburgh, who published the original data advocating the use of continuous pressure monitoring, recently reported the sensitivity and specificity of continuous monitoring.[38] Using a threshold for fasciotomy of a perfusion pressure sustained at less than 30 mm Hg for 2 hours or more, the calculated sensitivity of this method is 94%.[38] This sensitivity is far better than any single clinic examination finding, and establishes this technique as the best objective indication of the need for fasciotomy.

There are some pitfalls associated with the use of pressure measurements for decision making regarding fasciotomy in patients suspected of ACS. First, there is spatial variation in the pressure within a given compartment, with pressures highest within 5 cm of the fracture[39] and more centrally in the muscle.[40] However, there is no consensus on whether clinicians should obtain pressures near the fracture to obtain the highest pressure, or measure further away from the fracture to obtain a pressure that may be more representative of most of the compartment.[41] Second, there is error in the measurement, highlighted by a recent cadaveric study.[42] Using a standardized cadaver model of extremity compartment syndrome and a commercially available pressure monitor, 38 physicians were asked to measure intracompartment pressure. Correct technique was only used 31% of the time, and 30% of the measurements

were associated with a "catastrophic" error.[42] Furthermore, even when the correct technique was used, only 60% of the measurements made were accurate, with even greater inaccuracy when proper technique was not used.[42] Clinicians evaluating patients for ACS should be aware of these potential errors in the measurement of compartment pressures.

Another source of uncertainty in the determination of delta P is choosing what blood pressure value to use, especially if the patient is under general anesthesia. Kakar and colleagues[43] evaluated 242 patients undergoing tibial nailing, recording preoperative, intraoperative, and postoperative blood pressures. During surgery, there was a statistically significant decrease in diastolic blood pressure compared with preoperative values (average decrease, 18 mm Hg), whereas postoperative diastolic pressure was within 2 mm Hg of the preoperative value. Thus, use of intraoperative blood pressure measurements for calculation of perfusion pressure may give a spuriously low perfusion pressure and lead to unnecessary fasciotomy. These investigators recommend using preoperative blood pressure values to calculate perfusion pressure when patients are under general anesthesia, except when the patient is going to remain under anesthesia for several more hours.[43]

The presence of a known coagulopathy represents one of the only clear contraindications to fasciotomy, when doing a fasciotomy might cause exsanguination of the patient. A relative contraindication to fasciotomy is the late diagnosis of ACS, when muscle necrosis is already present. However, there are no validated methods to determine when it is too late, and substantial clinical experience is needed to make such a decision. In such settings, it is extremely important to document the history, examination findings, and the clinical reasoning that led to the choice to avoid fasciotomy in a given circumstance.

SURGICAL TECHNIQUE: DECOMPRESSIVE FASCIOTOMY

Decompressive fasciotomies must be done using 1 or more generous skin incisions with release of all constricting fascia within the involved muscle compartment. The specific locations of the incisions to be made and the anatomic structures that require release vary depending on the involved compartment. Fasciotomies must include an adequate skin incision in addition to the fascial release.

Double-incision Leg Fasciotomy

Fasciotomy of the 4 compartments of the lower leg is most safely done using 2 incisions: 1 medial and 1 lateral. The deep posterior compartment of the leg is released from the medial incision, whereas the lateral incision is used to decompress the anterior and lateral compartments. The superficial posterior compartment may be released from either incision. When the dual-incision technique is used, the intervening skin flap may be in jeopardy if there has been damage to the anterior tibial artery. If an anterior tibial artery injury is recognized before surgery, a single-incision 4-compartment release may be more appropriate (discussed later).

The lateral incision is made 2 to 3 cm lateral to the crest of the tibia (Fig. 1). Skin flaps are elevated by sharp dissection anteriorly and posteriorly, exposing the fascia of the anterior and lateral compartments. The lateral compartment fascia over the peroneal muscles is released. The lateral intermuscular septum that divides the anterior and lateral compartments and the superficial peroneal nerve are identified. In addition, the fascia over the anterior compartment is completely released. Alternatively, the fascia overlying the lateral compartment can be released followed by division of the intermuscular septum to decompress the anterior compartment. However, injury to the superficial peroneal nerve may be more likely with this technique.

The medial incision is made 1 to 2 cm posterior to the posteromedial border of the tibia. If the medial incision is placed too posteriorly, important perforating arterial branches to the skin from the posterior tibial artery may be damaged. The saphenous nerve and vein should be identified. The fascia of the gastrocnemius-soleus muscle complex should be completely released. The soleus bridge, representing the condensation of the anterior and posterior investing fascia of the soleus, should be released in order to identify and decompress the proximal portions of the flexor digitorum longus and posterior tibialis muscles.

These muscular components of the deep compartment should also be completely released.

Single-incision Leg Fasciotomy

Complete decompression of all 4 compartments of the lower leg may also be performed using a single long lateral incision extending from the neck of the fibula to the lateral malleolus. First, the anterior and lateral compartments are released as described earlier. The superficial posterior compartment (gastrocnemius-soleus complex) is easily released by elevating the skin posteriorly. Last, a parafibular approach is used to decompress the deep posterior leg compartment. In order to accomplish this, the peroneal muscles are retracted anteriorly, and the dissection is carried posterior to the fibula. With the lateral head of the gastrocnemius and soleus retracted posteriorly, the septum dividing the superficial and deep posterior compartments can be identified and released.

Thigh Fasciotomy

A long lateral thigh incision is made beginning at the distal aspect of the greater trochanter and extending to the lateral femoral epicondyle (Fig. 2). With deeper dissection, the iliotibial band is exposed and divided longitudinally. The vastus lateralis is identified and its investing fascia opened. Using a Cobb elevator, the muscle fibers of the vastus lateralis are teased off the lateral intermuscular septum, making sure to cauterize the perforating vessels as they are encountered. Make a 1-cm to 2-cm incision in the lateral intermuscular septum, and, using Metzenbaum scissors, extend it proximally and distally the length of the incision in order to decompress the posterior (hamstring) compartment. After the anterior and posterior compartments have been released from the lateral side, palpate or measure the pressure of the medial (adductor) compartment. If elevated, make a separate medial incision to release the adductor compartment.

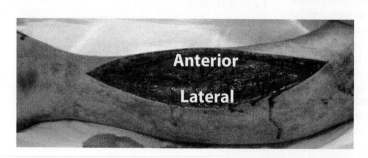

Fig. 1. A lateral leg fasciotomy showing the anterior and lateral compartments. Note the length of the fasciotomy wound, which should extend the length of the muscle compartment.

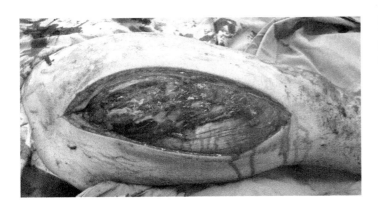

Fig. 2. A lateral thigh fasciotomy. The iliotibial band has also been incised, as has the fascia of the vastus lateralis.

Upper Extremity Fasciotomy

Compartment syndrome in the upper extremity can involve the upper arm, the forearm, and/or the hand. All involved compartments should be released. To decompress the upper arm, an anterior incision is made along the medial side of the biceps. The fascia of the biceps and underlying brachialis are easily released. If needed, the triceps are decompressed from a separate posterior incision. When needed, the anterior incision can be extended across the elbow and incorporated into a volar fasciotomy of the forearm. At the elbow, the incision should be carried across the flexor crease of the elbow in a zigzag fashion in order to avoid later contracture. The incision is then continued distally over the volar aspect of the forearm as needed. The volar incision should be carried along the medial border of the mobile wad toward the wrist (Fig. 3). The mobile wad, consisting of the brachioradialis and radial wrist extensors, is released. In order to decompress the forearm adequately, numerous potential sites of constriction need to be released, including the lacertus fibrosus, the muscle fascia, and the flexor retinaculum at the wrist. The fascia of the finger flexors, supinator, and pronator quadratus are all released as needed. A separate dorsal fasciotomy can be performed if needed using a midline approach between the extensor digitorum communis and the extensor carpi radialis brevis. The deep forearm is approached between the flexor carpi ulnaris and the flexor digitorum superficialis. It is necessary to divide 1 or 2 distal branches of the ulnar artery to the distal flexor digitorum superficialis in order to expose the pronator quadratus. In the middle third of the forearm, the ulnar neurovascular bundle is elevated with the flexor digitorum superficialis to expose the flexor digitorum profundus and the flexor pollicis longus. At the wrist, a standard carpal tunnel release is performed. If the forearm is also released, the incisions are carried across the wrist flexion crease in a zigzag fashion to avoid contracture. Injury to the palmar cutaneous branch of the median nerve must be avoided. In addition, if need be, the compartments of the hand can be released by release of the thenar, hypothenar, and interosseous muscles using short longitudinal incisions. Two dorsal hand incisions made between the second and third and the fourth and fifth metacarpals are sufficient to decompress the interosseous muscles.

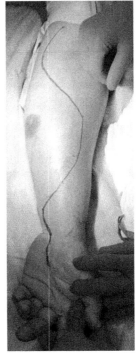

Fig. 3. The skin incision for a volar decompression of the forearm.

Foot Fasciotomy

The need for fasciotomy of the foot is controversial, with some experts believing that the morbidity of foot fasciotomy exceeds that of the sequelae of untreated foot compartment syndrome; namely clawing of the toes.

The foot has numerous functional compartments, but the abductor hallucis, interosseus muscles, and quadratus plantae (calcaneal compartment) are worthy of specific fasciotomy when compartment syndrome of the foot is diagnosed. As in the hand, the interosseous muscles are easily released with 2 dorsal longitudinal incisions. The abductor hallucis is released via a medial incision along the first ray, along with the quadratus plantae.

COMPLICATIONS AND THEIR MANAGEMENT

Fasciotomy is associated with its own set of complications, including the need for further surgery for delayed wound closure or skin grafting, pain, cosmetic problems, nerve injury, permanent muscle weakness, and chronic venous insufficiency (Fig. 4).[9,21,44–46]

Fasciotomy wounds should not be closed immediately because of the risk of causing increased muscle pressure and recurrent ACS. There is no consensus on when fasciotomies should be returned to the operating room for definitive closure. Typically, repeat debridement is performed every 48 to 72 hours when there is muscle necrosis until the wound remains stable. If viable tissues are found at the initial fasciotomy, it is the author's practice to wait 4 to 5 days before returning the patient to surgery for attempted wound closure.

POSTOPERATIVE CARE

Following fasciotomy, wound management is needed. In the past, wet-dry gauze bandages were used until the wound was deemed suitable for delayed closure or skin grafting. More recently, negative-pressure wound therapy (NPWT) has become a common method for managing a fasciotomy wound before closure. NPWT provides the theoretic benefits of removing fluid from the affected compartment, which reduces extracellular edema and helps to further reduce intracompartment pressures, as well as improving local blood flow and wound healing.[47] Advocates of NPWT suggest that wounds can be closed earlier and with less need for skin grafting.[48] However, NPWT was recently compared with the shoe-lace technique of wound closure in a randomized trial, with the NPWT technique being more expensive and associated with longer times to definitive wound closure.[49]

As described earlier, ACS is associated with increased costs of care, and these excessive costs are largely associated with the need for multiple follow-up surgical procedures, which are usually done in the hope of performing complete delayed wound closure. Weaver and colleagues[50] recently examined the utility of performing serial debridements, and found that when the fasciotomy wound could not be closed at the second surgery (first postfasciotomy procedure) it was rarely possible to perform complete delayed wound closure later. Skin grafting was also necessary in all wounds associated with open fractures.[50] These investigators suggest that immediate skin grafting should be done whenever the wound cannot be fully closed at the first repeat surgical session in order to reduce the length of hospitalizaion.[50]

OUTCOMES

Numerous articles document the efficacy of early fasciotomy[20,35,46,51,52] and the complications associated with late fasciotomy.[19,35] Despite the wide acceptance that compartment syndrome represents an orthopedic emergency,

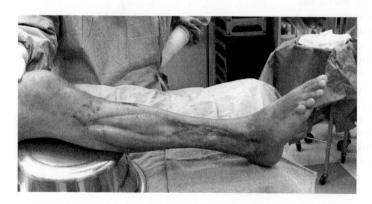

Fig. 4. A leg 2 years after undergoing a delayed fasciotomy for ACS after a tibial shaft fracture. There was significant muscle loss in the anterior and lateral compartments, as well as permanent nerve injury. Note the atrophic limb, clawing of the toes, and prior foot surgery for chronic ulceration. The photograph was taken before transtibial amputation.

Vaillancourt and colleagues[23] documented frequent delays both in the time from initial assessment to diagnosis and in the time from diagnosis to surgery. One study that specifically evaluated time from diagnosis to fasciotomy in 2 hospitals could not determine any statistical correlation between the time from diagnosis to fasciotomy and the presence of residual functional deficits.[53]

Sheridan and Matsen[35] found that fasciotomy performed within 12 hours of the onset of compartment syndrome, which they pragmatically defined as the first appearance of any clinical sign (motor weakness, stretch pain, or hypesthesia in the appropriate nerve), resulted in normal function in 68% of patients, compared with only 8% of those who had delayed fasciotomy.[35] In addition, patients undergoing late fasciotomy had a 10-fold increase in the rate of complications (4.5% vs 54%).[35]

SUMMARY

- Frequent clinical assessment of patients considered to be at risk for developing compartment syndrome, ideally using a structured checklist, remains the cornerstone of diagnosis. In alert patients, monitoring of limb swelling, pain (both at rest and with passive muscle stretching), and neurologic status provides clues to the onset of ACS. The clinical findings are of greatest utility when several findings are present together.
- When a patient is unconscious or otherwise not able to be clinically assessed at frequent intervals, then continuous measurement of intramuscular pressure within the anterior compartment is of benefit. Continuous pressure monitoring, using a threshold for fasciotomy of a perfusion pressure (diastolic pressure minus muscle pressure) sustained at less than 30 mm Hg for 2 hours, has a 93% positive predictive value for the diagnosis of ACS.
- Although based primarily on retrospective studies, the literature is convincing that, when compartment syndrome is going to occur, early fasciotomy can avoid myonecrosis or ischemic neuropathy. However, the challenges in diagnosis, and the fact that compartment syndrome does not begin at a well-defined point in time, make it impossible to draw specific conclusions about the optimum timing of fasciotomy.

REFERENCES

1. McQueen MM, Gaston P, Court-Brown CM. Acute compartment syndrome. Who is at risk? J Bone Joint Surg Br 2000;82:200–3.
2. Matsen FA. Compartment syndrome. A unified concept. Clin Orthop Rel Res 1975;113:8–14.
3. Ulmer T. The clinical diagnosis of compartment syndrome of the lower leg: are clinical findings predictive of the disorder? J Orthop Trauma 2002;16:572–7.
4. Mubarak SJ, Owen CA, Hargens AR, et al. Acute compartment syndromes: diagnosis and treatment with the aid of the wick catheter. J Bone Joint Surg Am 1978;60(8):1091–5.
5. Allen MJ, Stirling AJ, Crawshaw CV, et al. Intracompartmental pressure monitoring of leg injuries. An aid to management. J Bone Joint Surg Br 1985;67:53–7.
6. Badhe S, Baiju D, Elliott R, et al. The 'silent' compartment syndrome. Injury 2009;40:220–2.
7. Harrington P, Bunola J, Jennings AJ, et al. Acute compartment syndrome masked by intravenous morphine from a patient-controlled analgesia pump. Injury 2000;31:387–9.
8. Janzing HMJ, Broos PLO. Routine monitoring of compartment pressure in patients with tibial fractures: beware of overtreatment! Injury 2001;32:415–21.
9. Kashuk JL, Moore EE, Pinski S, et al. Lower extremity compartment syndrome in the acute care surgery paradigm: safety lessons learned. Patient Saf Surg 2009;3:11–6.
10. Prayson MJ, Chen JL, Hampers D, et al. Baseline compartment pressure measurements in isolated lower extremity fractures without clinical compartment syndrome. J Trauma 2006;60:1037–40.
11. Richards H, Langston A, Kulkarni R, et al. Does patient controlled analgesia delay the diagnosis of compartment syndrome following intramedullary nailing of the tibia? Injury 2004;35:296–8.
12. White TO, Howell GED, Will EM, et al. Elevated intramuscular pressures do not influence outcome after tibial fracture. J Trauma 2003;55:1133–8.
13. Williams PR, Russell ID, Mintowt-Czyz WJ. Compartment pressure monitoring–current UK orthopaedic practice. Injury 1998;29:229–32.
14. O'Toole RV, Whitney A, Merchant N, et al. Variation in diagnosis of compartment syndrome by surgeons treating tibial shaft fractures. J Trauma 2009;67:735–41.
15. Wall CJ, Richardson MD, Lowe AJ, et al. Survey of management of acute, traumatic compartment syndrome of the leg in Australia. J Trauma 2007;63:268–75.
16. Bhattacharyya T, Vrahas MS. The medical-legal aspects of compartment syndrome. J Bone Joint Surg Am 2004;86-A:864–8.

17. Vaillancourt C, Shrier I, Vandal A, et al. Acute compartment syndrome: how long before muscle necrosis occurs? CJEM 2004;6(3):147–54.
18. Finkelstein JA, Hunter GA, Hu RW. Lower limb compartment syndrome: course after delayed fasciotomy. J Trauma 1996;40:342–4.
19. Hope MJ, McQueen MM. Acute compartment syndrome in the absence of fracture. J Orthop Trauma 2004;18:220–4.
20. Prasarn ML, Ouellette EA, Livingstone A, et al. Acute pediatric upper extremity compartment syndrome in the absence of fracture. J Pediatr Orthop 2009;29:263–8.
21. Ritenour AE, Dorlac WC, Fang R, et al. Complications after fasciotomy revision and delayed compartment release in combat patients. J Trauma 2008;64:S153–62.
22. Shadgan B, Menon M, O'Brien PJ, et al. Diagnostic techniques in acute compartment syndrome of the leg. J Orthop Trauma 2008;22:581–7.
23. Vaillancourt C, Shrier I, Falk M, et al. Quantifying delays in the recognition and management of acute compartment syndrome. CJEM 2001;3: 26–30.
24. Crespo AM, Manoli A III, Konda SR, et al. Development of compartment syndrome negatively impacts length of stay and cost after tibia fracture. J Orthop Trauma 2015;29:312–5.
25. Schmidt AH. The impact of compartment syndrome on hospital length of stay and charges among adult patients admitted with a fracture of the tibia. J Orthop Trauma 2011;25: 355–7.
26. McQueen MM, Duckworth AD, Aitken SA, et al. Predictors of compartment syndrome after tibial fracture. J Orthop Trauma 2015;29:451–5.
27. Park S, Ahn J, Gee AO, et al. Compartment syndrome in tibial fractures. J Orthop Trauma 2009; 23:514–8.
28. Weinlein J, Schmidt AH. Compartment syndrome in tibial plateau fractures. Beware! J Knee Surg 2010;23:9–16.
29. Stark E, Stucken C, Trainer G, et al. Compartment syndrome in Schatzker type VI plateau fractures and medial knee fracture dislocations treated with temporary external fixation. J Orthop Trauma 2009;23:502–6.
30. Robinson CM, O'Donnell J, Will E, et al. Dropped hallux after the intramedullary nailing of tibial fractures. J Bone Joint Surg Br 1999;81:481–4.
31. Marcu D, Dunbar WH, Kaplan LD. Footdrop without significant pain as late presentation of acute peroneal compartment syndrome in an intercollegiate football player. Am J Orthop 2009;38(5): 241–4.
32. O'Sullivan MJ, Rice J, McGuinness AJ. Compartment syndrome without pain! Ir Med J 2002;95:22.
33. Whitesides TE, Haney TC, Morimoto K. Tissue pressure measurements as a determinant for the need for fasciotomy. Clin Orthop Rel Res 1975; 113:43–51.
34. McQueen MM, Court-Brown CM. Compartment monitoring in tibial fractures. The pressure threshold for decompression. J Bone Joint Surg Br 1996;78(1):99–104.
35. Sheridan GW, Matsen FA. Fasciotomy in the treatment of the acute compartment syndrome. J Bone Joint Surg Am 1976;58:112–5.
36. Øvre S, Hvaal K, Holm I, et al. Compartment pressure in nailed tibial fractures. A threshold of 30 mmHg for decompression gives 29% fasciotomies. Arch Orthop Trauma Surg 1998;118(1–2):29–31.
37. Schmidt AH. Continuous compartment pressure monitoring–better than clinical assessment? J Bone Joint Surg Am 2013;95(8):e52.
38. McQueen MM, Duckworth AD, Aitken SA, et al. The estimated sensitivity and specificity of compartment pressure monitoring for acute compartment syndrome. J Bone Joint Surg Am 2013;95:673–7.
39. Heckman MM, Whitesides TE, Grewe SR, et al. Compartment pressure in association with closed tibial fractures: the relationship between tissue pressure, compartment, and the distance from the site of the fracture. J Bone Joint Surg Am 1994;76:1285–92.
40. Nakhostine M, Styf JR, van Leuven S, et al. Intramuscular pressure varies with depth. The tibialis anterior muscle studied in 12 volunteers. Acta Orthop Scand 1993;64:377–81.
41. Harris IA, Kadir A, Donald G. Continuous compartment pressure monitoring for tibia fractures: does it influence outcome? J Trauma 2006;60:1330–5.
42. Large TM, Agel J, Holtzman DJ, et al. Interobserver variability in the measurement of lower leg compartment pressures. J Orthop Trauma 2015;316–21.
43. Kakar S, Firoozabadi R, McKean J, et al. Diastolic blood pressure in patients with tibia fractures under anesthesia: implications for the diagnosis of compartment syndrome. J Orthop Trauma 2007; 21:99–103.
44. Giannoudis PV, Nicolopoulos C, Dinopoulos H, et al. The impact of lower leg compartment syndrome on health related quality of life. Injury 2002;33:117–21.
45. Heemskerk J, Kitslaar P. Acute compartment syndrome of the lower leg: retrospective study on prevalence, technique, and outcome of fasciotomies. World J Surg 2003;27:744–7.
46. Mithoefer K, Lhowe DW, Vrahas MS, et al. Functional outcome after acute compartment syndrome of the thigh. J Bone Joint Surg Am 2006; 88:729–37.

47. Kakagia D. How to close a limb fasciotomy wound: an overview of current techniques. Int J Low Extrem Wounds 2015;14(3):268–76.

48. Yang CC, Chang DS, Webb LX. Vacuum-assisted closure for fasciotomy wounds following compartment syndrome of the leg. J Surg Orthop Adv 2006;15:19–23.

49. Kakagia D, Karadimas EJ, Drosos G, et al. Wound closure of leg fasciotomy: comparison of vacuum-assisted closure versus shoelace technique. A randomised study. Injury 2014;45(5):890–3.

50. Weaver MJ, Owen TM, Morgan JH, et al. Delayed primary closure of fasciotomy incisions in the lower leg: do we need to change our strategy? J Orthop Trauma 2015;29:308–11.

51. Rorabeck CH. The treatment of compartment syndromes of the leg. J Bone Joint Surg Br 1984; 66B:93–7.

52. Lagerstrom CF, Reed RL II, Rowlands BJ, et al. Early fasciotomy for acute clinically evident posttraumatic compartment syndrome. Am J Surg 1989; 158:36–9.

53. Cascio BM, Pateder DB, Wilckens JH, et al. Compartment syndrome: time from diagnosis to fasciotomy. J Surg Orthop Adv 2005;14: 117–21.

Treatment of Hip Dislocations and Associated Injuries
Current State of Care

Michael J. Beebe, MD[a], Jennifer M. Bauer, MD[b],
Hassan R. Mir, MD, MBA, FACS[a],*

KEYWORDS

• Hip dislocation • Acetabular fracture • Femoral head fracture • Irreducible dislocation
• Orthopedic emergency

KEY POINTS

• Time to initial hip relocation is considered an orthopedic emergency.
• Dislocations can be classified according to associated adjacent injuries, including acetabular, femoral head, and femoral neck fractures.
• Choice of open approach depends on visualization needed to treat associated hip injury.
• Complications include osteoarthritis, osteonecrosis, heterotopic ossification, and sciatic nerve palsy.
• Outcomes depend on the degree of initial trauma to the joint.

INTRODUCTION

Dislocations of the hip joint embody a wide range of injury patterns. However, all are similar in that they largely suggest a high-energy injury with considerable potential for both soft tissue and osseous injury. The hip is a stable, well-constrained ball-and-socket joint, requiring 40 to 60 kg (90–135 lb) of axial traction to simply distract and considerably more force to dislocate.[1] This high level of energy often results in associated injury to the labrum, femoral head, femoral neck, or acetabulum. These injuries may lead to protracted disability and dysfunction from complications such as osteoarthritis and avascular necrosis.

Hip dislocations have been reported in medical literature since the early nineteenth century[2]; however, the first considerable series of hip dislocations was published in 1938 by Funsten and colleagues[2] after the popularization of the ever-quickening automobile.[3] Subsequent series have revealed that most hip dislocations, 46% to 84%, occur secondary to traffic accidents, even with the advent of newer safety features.[3–9] The remaining minority most commonly occur because of falls, industrial accidents, or sporting injury.[4,6,10–12]

The treatment of hip dislocations, regardless of concomitant injury pattern, remains directed toward emergent reduction and attainment of a congruent joint through removal of imposing injured tissues and fixation of associated fractures. This article familiarizes readers with the classification, care, complications, and outcomes of hip dislocations and their associated injuries.

RELEVANT ANATOMY

Overall stability of the hip joint is reliant on the bony architecture and the joint's soft tissue

Disclosures: The authors received no funding and have no disclosures in relation to this current article.
[a] Orthopaedic Trauma Service, Florida Orthopaedic Institute, 5 Tampa General Circle, Suite 710, Tampa, FL 33602, USA; [b] Orthopaedic Surgery and Rehabilitation, Vanderbilt University, 1215 21st Avenue South, South Tower, Suite 4200, Nashville, TN 37232, USA
* Corresponding author.
E-mail address: hmir@floridaortho.com

constraints. As one of the most stable joints in the body, around 82% of the articular surface of the femoral head is enclosed by the bony acetabulum at neutral position.[13] This coverage is further extended by the labrum attached to the perimeter of the acetabulum. The labrum ensures that at least 50% of the femoral head is covered by the labral-acetabular complex in any position of hip motion.[14]

A thick capsule of longitudinally oriented fibers, save those circumferential fibers of the zona orbicularis, envelop the hip.[15] The longitudinal fibers thicken to form 3 distinct ligaments named for their origins and insertions.

- The iliofemoral ligament, also known as the Y ligament or ligament of Bigelow, arises in 2 distinct bands.[16] The medial band originates between the anterior-inferior iliac spine (AIIS) and the iliac portion of the acetabular rim and inserts on the distal intertrochanteric line. The lateral band originates superior to the medial band, closer to the AIIS, and runs oblique, downward, and lateral, to insert on the anterior greater trochanteric crest. Together, the 2 bands comprise the major static stabilizers of the hip in external rotation, whereas only the lateral band contributes significantly to stability in internal rotation.[16]
- The pubofemoral ligament originates from the anterior border of the superior pubic ramus and obturator crest with some fibers blending with the medial arm of the iliofemoral ligament and others wrapping inferiorly around the neck of the femur to insert on the posterior intertrochanteric crest. It controls external rotation in extension with contributions from the medial and lateral arms of the iliofemoral ligament.[16]
- Posteriorly, the ischiofemoral ligament is broad and less dense than the other two named ligaments, originating from the ischial portion of the acetabular rim and extending in an oblique and horizontal fashion to insert medial to the anterosuperior base of the greater trochanter and along the posterior intertrochanteric crest.[16]

In adults, the principal blood supply to the femoral head originates from the deep branch of the medial femoral circumflex artery. The chief division of the deep branch crosses posterior to the tendon of obturator externus and anterior to the superior gemellus, obturator internus, and inferior gemellus. It then perforates the hip capsule just cephalad to the insertion of the tendon of the superior gemellus and caudal to the tendon of piriformis before dividing into 2 to 4 superior retinacular arteries.[17] Lesser contributions arise through 2 central anastomoses (obturator and lateral femoral circumflex arteries [LFCA]) and 5 peripheral anastomoses (first perforating, LFCA, superior gluteal, inferior gluteal, and pudendal arteries).[17]

After confluence of nerves from nerve roots L4 to S3, the sciatic nerve exits the pelvis through the greater sciatic notch. Despite grossly appearing as a single nerve, the tibial and peroneal divisions have already formed before leaving the true pelvis. In around 83% of patients, the sciatic nerve courses anterior to the muscle body of the piriformis; however, in the remaining 17% the nerve varies from partially perforating the piriformis muscle body to coursing entirely posterior to the muscle body and any assortment in between.[18] This relationship may play a role in risk or protection of the nerve during dislocation, but is also an important consideration in surgical approach.

HISTORY, EXAMINATION, AND IMAGING
History
Patients with hip dislocations generally present after high-energy trauma. For this reason, patients often have distracting injuries or present in an obtunded state. It is imperative for physicians to recognize the signs and symptoms of a dislocation because delayed diagnosis in unconscious or obtunded patients can have serious results. Patients who are able to participate in an examination often complain of inability to move the lower extremity because of the semiconstrained position of the dislocated femoral head. They often endorse numbness or tingling in the affected extremity caused by neuropraxia of the sciatic nerve.

Examination
After appropriate Advanced Trauma Life Support (ATLS) management of a traumatized patient, examination of the lower extremity often reveals not only the presence of a dislocation but also the direction of dislocation.

- Patients with a posterior dislocation show hips that are flexed, adducted, and internally rotated.
- Patients with an anterior dislocation generally present with hips that are flexed, abducted, and strikingly externally rotated.

When a dislocation is present, after evaluation of limb position, careful attention must be paid to rule out both vascular and neurologic injury before any attempt at closed or open reduction. Sciatic nerve injuries are common, occurring in 10% to 15% of posterior dislocations.[4,10,12] The peroneal branch is most commonly affected, likely because of its posterior position and being tauter from tethering at the pelvis and the fibular neck.[19] However, tibial branch injury and even lumbosacral root avulsion have previously been reported with this injury.[20] Anterior dislocations have been, in rare cases, associated with vascular injury to the common femoral artery and vein.[19,21]

Urgent reduction may diminish the incidence or severity of nerve injury associated with dislocation, because time to reduction seems to be an independent risk factor for neurologic injury.[22] In a retrospective review of 106 posterior hip dislocations by Hillyard and Fox,[22] patients reduced at the initial presenting hospital (n = 69), at an average of 3.43 ± 1.59 hours from injury, showed a lower incidence (15% vs 30%, P = .0453) of major sciatic nerve injury (complete sciatic or peroneal motor deficit) than those transferred before reduction (n = 36), in whom reduction occurred at an average of 7.45 ± 4.15 hours from injury.[22]

The most common cause of dislocation, dashboard injury, often results in concurrent injury to the knee. Although it may be difficult to accurately examine the ligamentous stability of the knee before reduction, abrasion, ecchymosis, contusion, or laceration of the knee should alert physicians to the high likelihood of an associated injury to the knee.[23,24] Schmidt and colleagues[24] reported that up 89% of patients show signs of visible soft tissue injury on examination, whereas less than 10% of patients showed gross instability on ligamentous examination. Despite this, Schmidt and colleagues[24] reported that up to 93% of patients may have an injury to the ipsilateral knee on MRI, which is significantly higher than had previously been reported (24%–26%)[23,25] and should warrant absolute diligence in inspection of the knee during tertiary examination (Table 1).

Imaging

All patients with polytrauma, especially those presenting with altered mental status, should undergo a screening chest and pelvis radiograph performed in the trauma bay. The evaluating orthopedist must perform a careful and systematic evaluation of the anteroposterior (AP) pelvic radiograph for signs of lower lumbar injury,

	Number of Patients (n = 27)	Percentage of Patients
Table 1 Ipsilateral knee MRI findings associated with posterior hip dislocation		
Injury		
Posterior cruciate	5	19
Anterior cruciate	2	7
Collateral ligament	6	22
Meniscus	8	30
Extensor rupture	2	7
Periarticular fracture	4	15
Effusion	10	37
Bone bruise	9	33

Data from Schmidt GL, Sciulli R, Altman GT. Knee injury in patients experiencing a high-energy traumatic ipsilateral hip dislocation. J Bone Joint Surg Am 2005;87(6):1201–2.

pelvic ring or acetabular injury, hip dislocation, or proximal femoral fracture.

- In assessment of a possible dislocation, the femoral heads should appear symmetric in size with similar profiles of the greater and lesser trochanters. The femoral head should always clearly be positioned caudal to the acetabular dome.
- In an anterior dislocation, the dislocated femoral head appears larger than the contralateral hip, with a more en profile view of the lesser trochanter. Posterior dislocations most often display reduction in magnification of the dislocated femoral head, with a less apparent lesser trochanter profile.
- In a reduced hip, the joint space of the hip should show congruency throughout with a continuous flow to the Shenton lines. As always, vigilant assessment of the femoral neck must be performed to rule out a femoral neck fracture before an attempted reduction.

Once reduction has been obtained, repeat AP pelvis, Judet views, as well as AP and lateral hip radiographs should be carefully reviewed to confirm congruency of the joint and rule out concurrent fracture and fragment incarceration.

In general, it is our preference to forego computed tomography (CT) scanning before emergent reduction unless there is suspicion for a nondisplaced femoral neck fracture. After reduction, or in the case of an irreducible dislocation, CT should be routinely performed before any open procedure. In the case of an irreducible dislocation, CT scanning should be performed emergently to prevent delay of surgical intervention.

Based on the protocol by Tornetta and colleagues[26] for evaluation of the femoral neck following femoral shaft fracture, 2-mm or smaller cuts through the pelvis and femoral neck should be obtained to rule out occult femoral neck fracture. In patients undergoing dedicated pelvic CT ordered by the orthopedic team, our preference is to obtain 1-mm slices; however, in patients undergoing a standard chest, abdomen, and pelvis CT for trauma work-up, our institutional protocol is to perform 2-mm cuts through the pelvis. Thin slices through the pelvic region also allow appreciation of small osteochondral fragments that may remain in what may otherwise appear to be a congruently reduced joint on plain radiographs.[27] Ebraheim and colleagues[28] previously revealed that evaluation of CT images under soft tissue windowing in addition to standard bone windowing increased the identification of intraarticular osteochondral fragments.

The role of MRI after hip dislocation is not yet clearly defined. The sensitivity of MRI has, in small series, been shown to make it more accurate than CT in recognizing labral tears and osteochondral lesions associated with dislocation.[29,30] However, osseous evaluation on MRI is more difficult to interpret for surgical planning. MRI may play a role in evaluating a widened hip joint in the presence of a normal CT scan, decreasing radiation exposure in young or pregnant patients, or evaluating the hip joint in patients with worsening pain after resumption of ambulation and normal activities.[31]

CLASSIFICATION

Several classification systems have been developed for hip dislocations and their associated injuries. The first division in classification of hip dislocations is based on the direction of displacement of the femoral head in relation to the acetabulum.

Anterior Dislocations

Anterior dislocations account for around 9% to 24%[5,7,32] of all dislocations and patients generally present with a hip that is flexed, abducted, and externally rotated. This injury pattern was first classified by Epstein[33] into type A (superior/pubic) dislocations, wherein the femoral head dislocates superiorly abutting the superior pubic ramus, and type B (inferior/obturator) dislocations, in which the femoral head dislocates inferomedially into the obturator ring. Each type is further classified into 3 subtypes based on associated fractures. The mechanism for an anterior-inferior (type B) dislocation, as shown in a cadaveric model by Pringle and Edwards,[34] is that of simultaneous abduction, flexion, and external rotation of the hip, whereas anterior-superior (type A) dislocations occur secondary to extension and abduction.

Epstein[33] classification:

- Type A: pubic (superior)
  - 1: With no fracture (simple)
  - 2: With fracture of the head of the femur
  - 3: With fracture of the acetabulum
- Type B: obturator (inferior)
  - 1: With no fracture (simple)
  - 2: With fracture of the head of the femur
  - 3: With fracture of the acetabulum

Posterior Dislocations

The far more common posterior dislocation generally presents with a patient whose hip is flexed, adducted, and internally rotated. The most common mechanism is an axial load transmitted posteriorly through an adducted and flexed femur, such as occurs when a knee strikes the dashboard in a head-on collision.[2] Armstrong[35] first classified these injuries in 1948; however, several classification systems have since been proposed for this injury, with the most common being the Stewart and Milford[10] or Thompson and Epstein[32] classifications.

Armstrong[35] classification:
- Type I: simple dislocation
- Type II: dislocation with fracture of the acetabular rim
- Type III: dislocation with fracture of the acetabular floor
- Type IV: dislocation with fracture of the femoral head

Thompson and Epstein[32] classification:
- Type I: dislocation with or without minor fracture
- Type II: dislocation with large single fracture of the posterior acetabular rim
- Type III: dislocation with comminuted fracture of the rim of the acetabulum, with or without major fragment
- Type IV: dislocation with fracture of the acetabular rim and floor

- Type V: dislocation with fracture of the femoral head

Stewart and Milford[10] classification:
- Grade I: simple dislocation without fracture or with a chip from the acetabulum so small as to be of no consequence
- Grade II: dislocation with 1 or more large rim fragments, but with sufficient socket remaining to ensure stability after reduction
- Grade III: explosive or blast fracture with disintegration of the rim of the acetabulum, which produces gross instability
- Grade IV: dislocation with a fracture of the head or neck of the femur

Levin classification of posterior hip dislocations[14]:
- Type I: no significant associated fractures; no clinical instability after concentric reduction
- Type II: irreducible dislocation without significant femoral head or acetabular fractures (reduction must be attempted under general anesthesia)
- Type III: unstable hip after reduction or incarcerated fragments of cartilage, labrum, or bone
- Type IV: associated acetabular fracture requiring reconstruction to restore hip stability or joint congruity
- Type V: associated femoral head or femoral neck injury (fractures or impactions)

Orthopaedic Trauma Association (OTA)/ Arbeitsgemeinschaft für Osteosynthesefragen (AO) Classification[36]
- (A dislocation associated with an acetabular, femoral neck, or femoral head fracture should be coded with a fracture code and a dislocation code):
- 30–A1: anterior hip dislocation
- 30–A2: posterior hip dislocation
- 30–A3: medial or central hip dislocation
- 30–A4: obturator hip dislocation
- 30–A5: other hip dislocation

Management
Prompt reduction of the femoral head into the acetabulum is the first and foremost goal in treatment of a dislocated hip.

- Delayed reduction is thought to cause decreased blood flow to the femoral head, with several studies advocating reduction as soon as possible.[5,8,32]

- At our institution, every hip dislocation, other than those with a relative contraindication such as a femoral neck or shaft fracture, undergoes a closed reduction attempt under deep conscious sedation through propofol, in the emergency department (ED), before advanced imaging.
- Patients should be near or at the point of requiring respiratory assistance during the sedation for adequate muscle relaxation to create the least traumatic environment possible during reduction.
- Fluoroscopic imaging may be used during the reduction.
- Stable and concentric reductions are ranged through flexion-extension, adduction-abduction, and internal-external rotation while under sedation to determine degree of stability.
  ○ Dislocations with apparent interposed osteochondral fragments, those associated with large acetabular fractures affecting congruity, or those attendant to a femoral head fracture are placed into distal femur skeletal traction without ranging.
- Confirmatory AP pelvis and cross-table lateral hip radiographs are taken and the patient is then sent to the CT scanner to more accurately assess for periarticular fractures or intraarticular fragments.[27]
  ○ Judet, inlet, and outlet radiographs may also be obtained if CT scanning is not readily available, or reproduced from the CT scan with volume rendering techniques.
  ○ If CT scanning reveals intraarticular fragments not previously appreciated, skeletal traction is placed until surgery. Postreduction stability examination and CT scans are then used to determine the treatment plan.

If a hip is found to be irreducible in the ED, the patient is sent emergently to CT and then taken to the operating theater for reduction through either closed or open means.

CLOSED REDUCTION

Closed reduction is generally performed through disengagement of the femoral head from the acetabulum and recreation of the injury pattern with inline traction. Several reduction techniques, for the more common posterior dislocation, have been described.

The Bigelow[37] maneuver was initially described in 1870:

1. The patient is placed in the supine position.
2. The primary clinician provides an axial distraction force while an assistant applies a counterforce to the pelvis.
3. The hip is then adducted, internally rotated, and flexed to 90°.
4. With maintained traction, the hip is externally rotated, abducted, and extended as the femoral head reduces into the acetabulum.

Similar is the Allis[38] maneuver, first described in 1896:

1. The patient is placed in the supine position and the physician stands on the stretcher.
2. Inline traction is applied while an assistant applies counterpressure to the pelvis.
3. Reduction is obtained by traction, internal rotation, and then external rotation once the femoral hip clears the acetabular rim.

The Stimson[39] gravity technique was first described in 1883:

1. The patient is placed in the prone position with the injured leg hanging off the side of the bed.
2. The hip and knee are each brought to 90° of flexion.
3. The surgeon then applies an anteriorly directed force to the posterior calf.
4. Although effective, this method has the unfortunate requirement of placing the patient in the prone position, which makes airway management more difficult and may be impossible to perform safely in polytraumatized patients.

Skoff,[40] in 1986, described a new and unique method:

1. The patient is placed in the lateral decubitus position with the hip flexed to 100°.
2. The deformity is exaggerated with internal rotation of 45° and adduction of 45°.
3. Gravity-assisted distraction is allowed while an assistant applies direct posterior pressure to the femoral head as reduction occurs.

Howard[41] described a 3-person technique:

1. The patient is placed in the supine position.
2. The first assistant leans with both hands on the iliac crest of the affected side.

3. The second assistant flexes the femur to 90°, bringing the head of the femur from a posterosuperior position to lie directly posterior to the acetabulum.
4. The surgeon then grasps the proximal thigh and pulls the thigh laterally, allowing the head of the femur to clear the acetabular lip.
5. The second assistant applies longitudinal traction.

The senior author prefers to use the Rochester method, because it has proved to provide a controlled environment for single-person reduction[42]:

1. The patient is placed supine with the uninjured hip flexed to 45° and the knee flexed to 90°.
   a. The uninjured knee acts as a bolster for the arm that will be used as a pivot point for the reduction.
2. One of the surgeon's arms is placed underneath the injured knee, the forearm in the popliteal fossa of the injured leg, and the hand is placed on top of the uninjured knee, so that both knees and hips are now flexed.
3. The surgeon then grasps the ankle of the injured leg and, through downward pressure, the surgeon is able to pivot around the stable forearm to generate traction.
   a. The ankle can be used to provide internal and external rotation as needed.
4. Reduction is obtained by traction, internal rotation, and then external rotation once the femoral head clears the acetabular rim.

The East Baltimore lift reduction maneuver is similar to that of the Rochester method, but more appropriate for patients with contralateral leg disorder[43]:

1. The patient is placed supine and the injured hip and ipsilateral knee are placed in 90° of flexion.
2. The surgeon stands on the side of the dislocation with 1 assistant facing the surgeon on the opposite side of the bed.
3. The more proximal of the surgeon's arms, with respect to the patient, is positioned under the proximal calf of the injured leg with the surgeon's hand placed on the shoulder of the assistant across the table.
   a. The surgeon's other hand is used to control rotation of the distal leg.
4. The assistant then positions an arm in a similar fashion to that of the surgeon, crossing under

the proximal calf with the hand resting on the surgeon's shoulder.

a. A second assistant is used for stabilizing the pelvis.

5. The bed is lowered so that, as the surgeon and assistant stand from a squatted position, an anteriorly directed traction is applied to the hip.

After closed reduction of a hip in which the reduction is deemed concentric and stable, routine CT should be obtained to ensure no occult fracture is present.

OPERATIVE INTERVENTION
Approaches
Kocher-Langenbeck

Planning
- Positioning may be either lateral decubitus or prone, depending on surgeon preference.
- If in the lateral position, the injured leg may be draped free. An advantage of lateral positioning is the ability to test for hip stability following posterior repair and before wound closure.
- If in the prone position, distal femoral traction is generally placed and the leg is positioned into a traction table with the hip in extension and the knee flexed to slightly less than 90°.
- The use of a traction table may be optimal if an assistant is not available for traction.

Approach
- Incision is made along the posterior one-third of the femoral shaft to the tip of the trochanter and then curves posterosuperior at around a 45° angle to end 1 cm proximal to the posterior superior iliac spine (PSIS).
- The skin and subcutaneous fat are sharply dissected down to the tensor muscle, iliotibial band, and the gluteal fascia.
- The tensor fascia lata and iliotibial band are sharply divided in line with the fibers along the posterior aspect of the femoral shaft.
- After division of the gluteal fascia in line with the muscle fibers, gentle finger dissection can be used to split the muscle body of the gluteus maximus.
- Proximal extension is reached when the surgeon reaches the first crossing nerve fibers at approximately the halfway point between the PSIS and greater trochanter.

- The Charnley retractor is placed below this layer to optimize the view for the remainder of the procedure.
  - Iatrogenic injury to the sciatic nerve can occur if the posterior retractor arm is placed too deeply.
- The bursa overlying the greater trochanter is then excised to better visualize the short external rotators.
- The sciatic nerve is then identified and protected for the remainder of the procedure.
- A Hibbs retractor should be placed around the gluteus medius tendon for protection as the leg is internally rotated to put the short external rotators on stretch.
- The piriformis tendon is identified, tagged, and divided approximately 1 to 2 cm from its attachment to the femur to decrease risk of injury to the blood supply of the femoral head.
- The sciatic nerve should be readily visible at this point and should be assessed for contusion, hemorrhage, or laceration.
- The process is then repeated with a tagging suture placed into the obturator internus tendon with division of the superior and inferior gemelli and the obturator internus, again 1 to 2 cm from their insertion.
  - The gemelli and the obturator internus provide protection for the sciatic nerve because of its course along the posterior aspect of this muscle group.
- In most patients, the sciatic nerve is found anterior to the piriformis after it is released.
- The next caudal muscle is the body of the quadratus femoris, which must be left intact to prevent injury to the medial femoral circumflex artery running along its superior border.
- At this point, a sciatic nerve retractor is placed.
- By following the short external rotators, the surgeon may easily find both the greater (piriformis) and lesser (obturator internus) sciatic notches.
- Placement of the retractor in the lesser sciatic notch allows for protection of the sciatic nerve with the obturator internus muscle belly.
- A second retractor may be placed into the greater sciatic notch, but caution must be exercised to limit the risk of injury to the sciatic nerve and the superior gluteal neurovascular bundle.

- The posterior capsule and acetabular rim are now within view.
- In the setting of a posterior wall fracture, further disruption of the capsule must be avoided to prevent devascularization of the acetabular wall fragment. The labrum and capsule are typically torn and detached caudally by the injury.
- If the acetabular wall remains intact, the capsule is most likely to be torn from the dislocation. Should the capsule remain intact or require further dissection, capsulotomy must be performed at the acetabular origin to prevent injury to the vascular supply of the femoral head.
- Care must be taken to avoid injury to the labrum during release.
- Once exposed, the femoral head may require further distraction through either the fracture table or an assistant.
- Placement of a Steinmann pin into the lateral aspect of the proximal femur can help with pure lateral distraction.
- It is rare to require complete redislocation of the femoral head and, if this is the case, it is our preference to proceed with a surgical dislocation, as discussed later.

Surgical dislocation/digastric osteotomy

Planning

- Surgical dislocation as described by Ganz and colleagues[44] provides exceptional visualization of the femoral head and acetabulum in cases in which both anterior and posterior access is required.
- The patient is positioned in the lateral decubitus position.
- A sterile bag is placed on the side opposite the surgeon in which to place the leg during dislocation.

Approach

- Incision is made along the posterior one-third of the femoral shaft to the tip of the trochanter, and it then curves posterosuperiorly at around a 45° angle to end 1 cm proximal to the PSIS.
- The skin and subcutaneous fat are sharply dissected down to the tensor muscle, iliotibial band, and the gluteal fascia.
- The tensor fascia lata and iliotibial band are sharply divided in line with the fibers along the posterior aspect of the femoral shaft.
- The leg is then internally rotated and the posterior border of the gluteus medius tendon is identified.

- A mark is then made from the posterior superior edge of the greater trochanter to the posterior border of the vastus lateralis ridge.
- An oscillating saw is then used to perform the osteotomy along this line and in a sagittal plane through the femur.
  - Some surgeons prefer to drill for fixation before completion of the osteotomy.
- At the proximal aspect of the osteotomy, the exit point should be just anterior to the posteriormost insertion of the medius tendon and distally the vastus lateralis attachment should remain intact to the wafer.
  - This technique allows preservation of the medial femoral circumflex artery, which becomes intracapsular at the level of the superior gemellus muscle.[17,44]
  - The osteotomy is correctly placed when only a small portion of the piriformis requires release from the free fragment.
- The vastus lateralis is then freed from the lateral and anterior proximal femur for mobilization of the fragment.
- The gluteus minimus tendon is separated from the piriformis and underlying capsule.
- There is a constant anastomosis between the inferior gluteal artery and the medial femoral circumflex running along the inferior border of the piriformis that is preserved and may be used to trace to the medial femoral circumflex.
- A Z-shaped capsulotomy is performed starting with an anterolateral incision in line with the neck. The capsular incision is then carried down the anterior aspect of the neck just before the vastus ridge. The posterior limb is placed immediately adjacent to the acetabular insertion.
- Once the capsulotomy is complete, the hip is dislocated through flexion and external rotation as the leg is brought into a sterile bag on the side of the table opposite the surgeon.
- By controlling the leg, the surgeon now has full access to the acetabulum and femoral head.
- After completion of operative fixation, the capsule is repaired and the osteotomy is fixed into anatomic position with two 3.5-mm cortical screws with or without washers.

Postoperative

- ○ Active abduction should be avoided through touchdown weight bearing for the first 6 to 8 weeks, regardless of limitations based on fixation or lack thereof (**Fig. 1**).

Smith-Peterson approach

Planning

- ○ The patient is positioned supine with the operative leg draped free either on a radiolucent flat top table or on a fracture table.
- ○ Draping should include the entire ipsilateral flank and leg to allow extension in either direction when necessary.

Approach

- ○ The planned incision begins just lateral to the anterior-superior iliac spine (ASIS), then curves down in line with the lateral border of the sartorius to end approximately 10 cm inferior to the ASIS.
  - ■ This procedure may require extension in either direction for further exposure.
- ○ Subcutaneous flaps are raised medially and laterally, aiming to identify the fascia over the tensor fasciae latae muscle belly.
- ○ The interval between the sartorius and the tensor fasciae latae is identified distally and traced proximally, incising sharply in line with the fascial fibers while taking care to identify and avoid direct trauma to the lateral femoral cutaneous nerve, which courses through the fascia.
- ○ Finger dissection of the plane between the tensor and sartorius is then performed, followed deeper blunt dissection in the plane between the rectus femoris and gluteus medius.

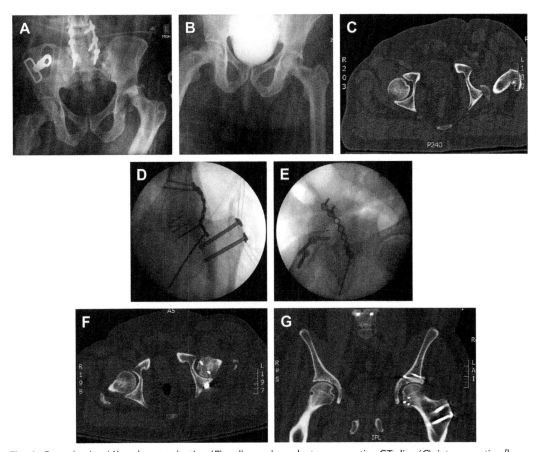

Fig. 1. Prereduction (A) and postreduction (B) radiographs, select preoperative CT slice (C), intraoperative fluoroscopic images (D, E), and select postoperative CT slices (F, G) of a dislocation resulting in both a posterior wall fracture and a femoral head fracture. Rather than perform 2 separate approaches for the injury, a surgical dislocation was performed for fixation through a single approach.

○ The ascending branches of the lateral femoral circumflex artery are encountered in this deeper interval and must be either well cauterized or suture ligated to avoid excessive bleeding.

○ The fat overlying the capsule and iliocapsularis muscle fibers may be excised.

○ The rectus may be released from the anterior capsule to improve visualization.

○ Retraction of the rectus femoris and iliopsoas medially and gluteus medius allows visualization of the capsule.

○ A longitudinal or T-shaped incision is then made along the anterior capsule with care to avoid labral injury.

  ■ The vertical limb of the T is made first in line with the femoral neck, followed by the cross portion of the T adjacent to the labrum.

  ■ Adduction and external rotation of the hip place the capsule on stretch, allowing an easier capsulotomy.

○ At this point, the surgeon should have optimal visualization of the femoral neck and anterior head.

  ■ Dislocation of the hip may be performed through external rotation for further visualization of the femoral head or debridement of the joint.

Postoperative

○ Postoperatively, single-dose radiation or nonsteroidal prophylaxis may be considered because Swiontkowski and colleagues[45] showed that although treatment of femoral head fractures through the anterior approach did not alter the rate of avascular necrosis, the risk of heterotopic ossification was significantly increased.

Dislocation and Fracture-dislocation Categories

Concentric and stable reduction

In the past, stable and concentric reductions with normal advanced imaging have been treated without any type of surgical intervention, unless pain continued or worsened with prolonged conservative treatment.[14] Recent data by several groups have shown that, even with a normal CT scan or MRI, patients may have retained loose bodies within the hip joint.[46–48]

○ Mullis and Dahners noted that 25 of 36 patients (69%) in their series had a loose body on arthroscopic evaluation.[49] Seven

of the 9 patients (78%) who had a negative CT had an intraarticular loose body.

○ Yamamoto and colleagues,[47] in a series of 11 hips, found that 7 joints (64%) had arthroscopic fragments not noted on CT.

○ Wylie and colleagues[46] noted that 2 of 12 patients, less than the age of 25 years, had previously undiagnosed chondral loose bodies on arthroscopy, whereas 8 of 12 (67%) had some type of loose body.

  ■ However, they noted that although their patients had a mix of MRI and CT scans before arthroscopy, the 2 with previously undiagnosed chondral fragments did not have MRI before the procedure, which may have allowed visualization through advanced imaging.

Given the current evidence that a hip joint with a concentric and stable reduction with normal postreduction advance imaging may have retained intraarticular loose bodies, it is imperative that surgeons have a frank discussion with their patients regarding the possibility of retained loose bodies. In patients with an otherwise normal hip joint free of preexisting arthrosis and with a normal CT scan, consideration can be given to performing either thin-slice MRI or arthroscopy for evaluation of loose bodies. If loose bodies are present, arthroscopic debridement may then be pursued.

Eccentric or unstable reduction

After closed reduction of a hip, it is crucial that the surgeon immediately obtains radiographic imaging to determine the concentricity of the reduction, because an eccentric reduction greatly alters management. If postreduction imaging shows a concentric reduction, preferably while still under conscious sedation, the hip should be sequenced through a range of motion to determine stability.

○ In the case of a posterior dislocation, emphasis should be placed on flexion, adduction, and internal rotation with an axial load.

○ In an anterior dislocation, extension, adduction, and external rotation place the hip at its point of maximal instability.

In the context of a concentric reduction with continued instability on examination, the surgeon has several options. Our preference is to proceed with a postreduction CT scan to evaluate any unrecognized osseous injuries or small, incarcerated fragments that may not be initially recognized on plain radiographs.

- o If CT shows any osseous injury that could be correlated with continued instability, open reduction and fixation should be performed, as described later in this article.
- o If the CT is within normal limits, then MRI may be warranted.
  - As mentioned earlier, the sensitivity of MRI has, in small series, been shown to be greater than that of CT in recognizing labral tears and osteochondral lesions associated with dislocation and thus surgeons may choose to proceed directly with MRI and limit radiation exposure to the patient.[29,30]

The patient may also be taken to the operating theater for a stress examination under anesthesia using fluoroscopic imaging.[50] If significant hip instability is present, then an open approach with joint exploration and posterior capsulolabral repair may be performed. Although several investigators have attributed the importance of posterior wall fracture fragment size to the presence or absence of recurrent instability,[51–55] less inquiry has gone into the subject of instability after posttraumatic labral injury. Thus case reports and small case series comprise the breadth of evidence with regard to labral repair and its efficacy in diminishing recurrent instability.[56–58]

Nonetheless, the labrum has been shown to decrease both stress and strain on the hip joint and chondral surface, playing an important role in maintaining fluid film lubrication and likely in the prevention of future arthritic change.[59–61] Minor labral injuries or capsular disruptions may be treated with a hip-knee orthosis limited to the stable arc of motion and possible delayed surgical intervention; however, complete disruption of the circumferential fibers of the labrum may warrant immediate open or arthroscopic repair.[14,62]

Presence of intraarticular fragments on CT or MRI always warrants skeletal traction followed by urgent removal, because these will rapidly degrade the chondral surface if left in place. If large enough to be returned and fixed into position, an open approach that places the fragment's origin in direct view will best serve the surgeon. If too small to replace, removal may be performed through either an arthroscopic or an open approach.[62–64] Note that arthroscopy should not be performed in cases with a known or suspected acetabular fracture, even when nondisplaced, because extravasation of fluid into the intrapelvic region can result in life-threatening abdominal compartment syndrome.[65–67] Rarely, traction alone does not allow the surgeon to retrieve the fragment and a surgical dislocation may be warranted to allow full access to the entirety of the acetabulum and femoral head.[44,68]

Irreducible simple dislocation

Simple dislocations are most often reducible through closed means under appropriate sedation; however, if irreducible, it is imperative that the patient be taken urgently to the operating theater. An expeditious preoperative CT scan is warranted, because this may reveal a small, otherwise unrecognized fracture, which may change operative planning. Once under general anesthesia and with complete paralysis, the surgeon may again decide to attempt closed reduction. However, physicians must be aware that multiple attempts at closed reduction may result in further traumatic injury to the chondral surface of the femoral head, in contrast with a controlled open reduction.

There have been several reports on irreducible dislocation without apparent fracture due to a variety of causes. Most previous reports place the rate of irreducible dislocation, without fracture, at around 2% to 6%.[9,32,69–74]

Once the surgeon decides to proceed with open reduction, there are several possible approaches. Without a fracture present, it is sensible to choose an approach that places the dislocated femoral head in direct view.

- o Posterior dislocations are treated best with a Kocher-Langenbeck approach.
- o Anterior dislocations are best treated through a Watson-Jones, Hardinge, or Smith-Peterson approach.

The surgeon must take great care during the approach, because the still-dislocated femoral head will distort normal anatomy, often displacing the neurovascular structures into the surgical field.

Once the chosen approach is complete, the surgeon should use the opportunity of the dislocation to examine the exposed acetabulum and femoral head for nondisplaced fracture or marginal impaction.

- o Loose bodies or interposed tissue should be removed from the acetabulum.
- o Osteochondral fragments, if large enough, should undergo reduction and fixation.

○ The acetabulum should then be thoroughly irrigated before reduction.

Several investigators have reported on the imposing structures preventing closed reduction of posterior hip dislocations.

- Slätis and Latvala[71] reported 2 cases, one in which the piriformis muscle was found to be twisted around the femoral neck, blocking the entrance to the acetabulum, and a second in which the obturator internus, the gemellus superior, and the gemellus inferior muscles had been torn from their respective origins and filled the acetabulum.
- In possibly a more common scenario, Hunter[9] reported a case of a buttonhole tear of the posterior capsule entrapping the femoral head.
- In the 3 cases of irreducible dislocation reported by Canale and Manugian,[69] the femoral head was buttonholed through the capsule in 2 and the piriformis muscle became displaced across the acetabulum in 1.
  ○ They further reported on 6 cases of nonconcentric reduction caused by an inverted labrum in 3, an osteocartilaginous body in 2, and both in 1 (Fig. 2).

After the hip is reduced, fluoroscopic imaging should be obtained, similar to a simple reduction, to confirm a concentric reduction before assessing stability. It is common for an osteochondral fragment from either the acetabulum or femoral head, hidden because of limited visibility from the approach, to become incarcerated in the joint after reduction. In our experience, expeditiously obtaining a CT scan before open reduction decreases the likelihood of a fragment being missed and limits the possibility of performing an approach where such a fragment is inaccessible for reduction and fixation.

After the hip is concentrically reduced, the surgeon should take the joint through a range of motion. In the case of posterior dislocation, focus should remain on flexion, adduction, and internal rotation. In an anterior dislocation, extension, adduction, and external rotation is the position of instability. Once in the position of maximum stress, axial force should be applied to the thigh to determine absolute stability. Instability must be immediately investigated before closure. Repair of capsular injury or labral tears is warranted.

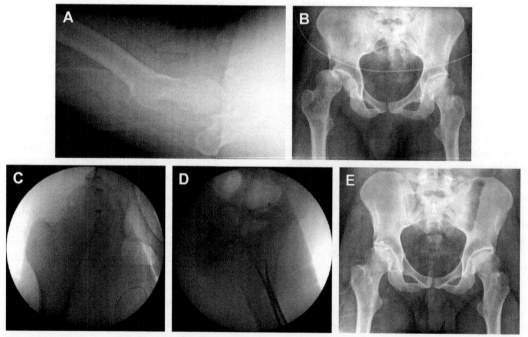

Fig. 2. Prereduction radiographs (A, B), intraoperative fluoroscopic images (C, D), and a postoperative radiograph (E) of a dysplastic hip in a patient who presented with an irreducible dislocation. Open reduction showed interposition of the labrum and posterior capsule into the acetabulum, which was subsequently repaired using suture anchor fixation.

Dislocation with acetabular fracture

The mechanism of injury for isolated acetabular fractures is similar to that of isolated hip dislocations, thus dislocations of the hip may result in a variety of acetabular fracture patterns.

The 2-column concept of acetabular morphology and fracture classification was introduced by Letournel[75] and is still the most popular classification system.

- In brief, the acetabulum is supported by an inverted Y formed by 2 columns of bone.
  - The anterior column tracks obliquely from the anterior part of the superior iliac crest to the pubic symphysis.[75] It is formed by the symphysis pubis, the superior pubic ramus, the anterior acetabular wall, the anterior half of the acetabulum, the anterior half of the quadrilateral plate, and the anterior ilium.[14]
  - The posterior column descends from the angle of the greater sciatic notch to the ischial tuberosity and contains the entire posterior wall, the posterior acetabulum, the inferior aspect of the greater sciatic notch, the ischial spine, the entire lesser sciatic notch, and the posterior half of the quadrilateral surface.[14,75]
- Fracture patterns are divided into elementary and associated patterns.
  - Elementary fracture patterns are those in which 1 part or all of 1 column has been detached, with the exception of the pure transverse, which was included in this category by virtue of its purity.[75]
  - The associated patterns are those that include a combination of at least 2 of the elementary patterns (Table 2).

As in similar dislocation events, emergent reduction is first priority, and can most often be achieved in the ED with conscious sedation. Once reduction is achieved, skeletal traction should be considered to ensure that the hip remains reduced. Without traction, the hip often either subluxates or fully dislocates because of the loss of stability within the acetabulum.

After reduction is achieved, a CT scan allows the surgeon to assess the fracture pattern. Judet views may allow similar assessment, depending on surgeon preference. Although faux Judet views obtained through CT reconstruction may prove both less time consuming and easier to comfortably obtain, the act of rolling the patient to each side effectively provides a stress examination for the hip, thus faux Judet views do not provide an exact facsimile of true Judet views. Once the fracture pattern is determined, this guides the surgeon in the necessary approach for operative fixation. Most fractures can be treated through a single approach; however, some fractures require the surgeon to approach the fracture from both an anterior and posterior approach[76,77] (Table 3).

The most common fracture pattern in general and the most common pattern associated with a hip dislocation is an isolated fracture of the posterior wall.[75,78] In determining whether fixation is required, surgeons must assess the stability of the hip after reduction. Although fragment size may help guide assessment of stability, previous literature has shown that, even in patients with hips deemed stable (<20% wall involvement) on CT, dynamic stress under anesthesia shows a significant number of erroneous results based on CT alone.[51,54,55,79,80] Thus, in most patients with a posterior wall fracture, examination under anesthesia is warranted. Most isolated posterior wall fractures can be treated through a standard Kocher-Langenbeck approach. Those fractures that extend to the superior dome may require osteotomy of the trochanter to further translate the abductors anterior and access the dome segment[81,82] (Fig. 3).

Table 2 Acetabular fracture patterns as described by Letournel	
Elementary Fracture Patterns	**Associated Fracture Patterns**
Posterior wall	Associated both column
Posterior column	Transverse + posterior wall
Anterior wall	T shaped
Anterior column	Anterior column/wall + posterior hemitransverse
Pure transverse	Posterior column + posterior wall

Data from Letournel E. Acetabulum fractures: classification and management. Clin Orthop Relat Res 1980;(151):81–106.

Table 3
Standard acetabular approaches and their indications

Approach	Indications
Anterior intrapelvic + Lateral (first) window of ilioinguinal or Full ilioinguinal	Anterior wall Anterior column Most associated both column Anterior column/wall + posterior hemitransverse Transverse with high posterior column T shaped with high posterior column
Kocher-Langenbeck	Posterior wall Posterior column Posterior column + posterior wall Most transverse + posterior wall Most pure transverse Most T shaped
Dual approach	Transverse with displaced anterior column after posterior reduction T shaped with displaced anterior column after posterior reduction Associated both column with posterior comminution

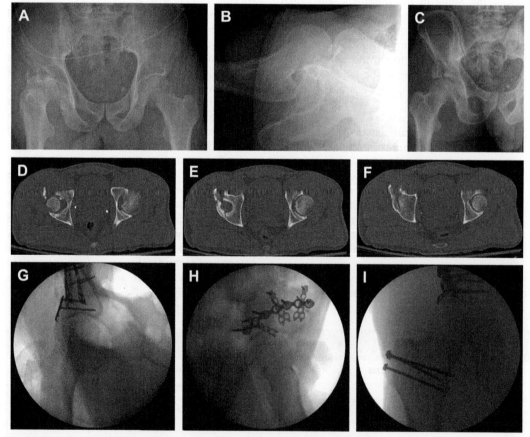

Fig. 3. Prereduction (*A*, *B*) and postreduction (*C*) radiographs, select preoperative CT slices (*D–F*), and intraoperative fluoroscopic images (*G–I*) of a dislocation resulting in a high posterior wall fracture extending anteriorly around to the AIIS. Reduction and internal fixation required a digastric osteotomy for visualization of the superior acetabulum.

Isolated anterior wall fractures are the least common of all types, but may occur in association with an anterior dislocation. Surgeons must be careful not to confuse an anterior wall fracture with a stable pubic root fracture that extends into the anterior acetabulum. True anterior wall fractures, although rare, may prove difficult to access. Access often requires either developing the middle (second) window of the ilioinguinal approach or an anterior intrapelvic approach with an ASIS osteotomy.[83,84]

It is likely that the fracture-dislocation with the worst outcome is the so-called medial dislocation (OTA/AO 30–A3), in which the femoral head punches through the quadrilateral plate into the true pelvis. Most fractures in this pattern occur secondary to lateral hip loading in elderly patients.[85,86] The incidence of marginal impaction is higher in elderly patients, as is the incidence of postoperative arthrosis even with anatomic reduction.

At presentation, patients should be placed into skeletal traction and reduction of the femoral head into a more anatomic position should be attempted through distal and lateral traction. It is common for the femoral head to become incarcerated within the pelvis as the quadrilateral plate closes down around the femoral neck. If this occurs, emergent reduction must be performed unless the surgeon plans to proceed with a combined arthroplasty procedure.[87] After the hip is reduced, or in the case of an irreducible hip, CT scan should be obtained before operative treatment. Most of these fractures are best treated through an anterior intrapelvic and lateral window approach to optimally visualize the quadrilateral plate. However, because of the poor quality of bone in this group of patients, comminution of the posterior column is frequently encountered, which may require a dual approach for adequate reduction and fixation.[76]

Dislocation with femoral head fracture
Femoral head fractures are less common than acetabular fractures after hip dislocation, with around 5% to 15% of hip dislocations presenting with an associated femoral head fracture.[7,88–91] Although only 10% of femoral head fractures are associated with an anterior dislocation, around 70% of anterior dislocations occur in conjunction with a femoral head fracture.[92,93] Regardless of the direction in which the hip dislocates, femoral head fracture incidence has steadily increased, likely secondary to improvements in both automobile safety and resuscitation technique.[91]

With roughly 70% of the articular surface of the femoral head engaging in load transfer, loss of congruency of the articular surface either through fracture displacement or impaction can lead to significant changes in the load through the hip joint.[94] It is thus imperative to achieve anatomic congruity of the articular surface.

Although several classification systems have been developed, 2 main femoral head fracture-dislocation taxonomies have been widely used: the Pipkin and Brumback classifications. The Pipkin classification system is more widely used, classifying fractures based on location and associated fractures. The Brumback classification system is more descriptive and thus ideal for use in clinical research.

Pipkin[95] classification system:
- Type 1: dislocation with fracture of the femoral head caudad to the fovea capitis femoris
- Type 2: dislocation with fracture of the femoral head cephalad to the fovea capitis femoris
- Type 3: type 1 or 2 injury associated with fracture of the femoral neck
- Type 4: type 1 or 2 injury associated with fracture of the acetabular rim

Brumback[92] classification system:
- Type 1: posterior hip dislocation with fracture of the femoral head involving the inferomedial (non–weight-bearing) portion of the femoral head
  - Type 1A: with minimum or no fracture of the acetabular rim and stable hip joint after reduction
  - Type 1B: with significant acetabular fracture and hip joint instability
- Type 2: posterior hip dislocation with fracture of the femoral head involving the superomedial (weight-bearing) portion of the femoral head
  - Type 2A: with minimum or no fracture of the acetabular rim and stable hip joint after reduction
  - Type 2B: with significant acetabular fracture and hip joint instability
- Type 3: dislocation of the hip (unspecified direction) with femoral neck fracture
  - Type 3A: without fracture of the femoral head
  - Type 3B: with fracture of the femoral head

- Type 4: anterior dislocation of the hip with fracture of the femoral head
  - Type 4A: indentation type: depression of the superolateral surface of the femoral head
  - Type 4B: transchondral type: osteocartilaginous shear fracture of the weight-bearing surface of the femoral head
- Type 5: central fracture-dislocation of the hip with femoral head fracture

Initial management of patients with a femoral head fracture is similar to that of patients with any other hip dislocation in that the first goal is reduction of the femoral head within the acetabulum. In patients in whom closed reduction is possible in the ED, it is our preference to perform closed reduction before obtaining a CT scan.

A unique, uncommon variation is the irreducible dislocation associated with femoral head fractures.[12] In this dislocation, the proximal femur is docked against the supra-acetabular lateral ilium and the capsule and/or labrum blocks any attempt at closed reduction. Iatrogenic femoral neck fracture may result when excessive force is used to attempt to overcome this mechanical block. Irreducible hip dislocations warrant emergent open reduction.

Typical hip position on presentation for each main category includes:

- Anterior: hip flexed, abducted, externally rotated
- Posterior: hip flexed, adducted, internally rotated
- Irreducible: less flexion, neutral rotation, obvious shortened length[12]

It is our preference to place patients with femoral head fractures in skeletal traction, if the fragment is not in anatomic position after reduction. This method theoretically limits the amount of further damage to both the femoral head and acetabular chondral surfaces before surgical intervention.

Pipkin type I fractures with near-anatomic position (<2-mm incongruity) in conjunction with a stable and congruent hip joint can potentially be treated nonoperative and still obtain good to excellent results.[45,91] It is our preference to confirm stability with an examination under anesthesia with fluoroscopy. Pipkin type II to IV fractures, hips with displaced or incarcerated fragments, and fractures in the setting of an unstable hip require operative intervention.

Investigators have used nearly every described approach to the hip for femoral head fractures; however, 3 main approaches are used more than the others: the Kocher-Langenbeck (posterior), Smith-Petersen (anterior), and surgical dislocation (digastric flip). Epstein and colleagues[88] thought that, because the femoral head blood supply had already been violated along the posterior aspect of the hip from a posterior dislocation, an anterior approach was contraindicated for concern of further damage to the anterior blood supply. This theory was tested by Swiontkowski and colleagues,[45] who retrospectively reviewed 29 patients, 12 of whom had an anterior approach and 12 of whom had a posterior approach, and there was no difference in the avascular necrosis rate between groups. There was significantly less blood loss and shorter operative time in the anterior group; however, the anterior group also saw a higher rate of heterotopic ossification. The findings, with regard to the lack of difference in the rate of avascular necrosis, have been reinforced by subsequent studies.[91,96,97] In contrast, Stannard and colleagues[97] found that the posterior approach showed an avascular necrosis rate 3.2 times higher than that of the anterior approach in caring for posterior dislocations.

In the past, fragment excision was a popular method of treating femoral head fractures, as long as the fragment comprised less than one-third of the femoral head.[89,91,98] Marchetti and colleagues,[96] in a review of 33 patients, showed that patients who underwent excision had an insignificant improvement in outcomes compared with open reduction and internal fixation (80% vs 53% good results). Similarly, Stannard and colleagues,[97] in a retrospective review of 22 patients who underwent either fixation or excision, showed that both groups had poor, but overall equivalent, outcomes regardless of treatment. Both groups had an average Short Form-12 physical component score of 40 at a mean of 24 months' follow-up.

In our experience, the decision to excise or fix a fragment is determined by the position, extent, and comminution of the fragment. Pipkin type 1 fractures with small fragments or those with significant comminution to the point of preventing adequate fixation are generally excised. Park and colleagues[99] recently evaluated 59 patients treated with either excision or open reduction and internal fixation of the fracture fragment. In patients with large infrafoveal fragments, the patients who underwent operative fixation of the fragment had a greater chance at an excellent or good outcome (85.7% vs 60.0%; P = .05). In the case of a Pipkin type II fracture (suprafoveal fragment), or a Pipkin III to IV fracture with a suprafoveal fragment, attempt at operative fixation is nearly always warranted, unless arthroplasty is planned.

After determination of the type of fracture, location, and comminution, if surgeons choose to attempt operative fixation, they should choose an approach that offers the best access to the fragment's normal anatomic location.

- In the case of an anterior fracture, the Smith-Peterson approach usually provides the best visualization.
- A posterior fracture is best managed through the Kocher-Langenbeck approach.
  - The benefit of the Kocher-Langenbeck approach is that it can easily be converted to a surgical hip dislocation, if necessary to access the central or anterior head.[100]
- In the case of a Pipkin III fracture, a femoral head fracture with associated femoral neck, the surgeon should plan to stabilize the femoral neck before attempting reduction and fixation of the femoral head.
  - For basicervical femoral neck fractures, the Watson-Jones approach may provide enough visualization for open reduction and, at the same time, placement of a sliding hip screw (SHS) through the same approach, which is the optimal implant in a basicervical fracture.
  - However, for more medial fractures, a Smith-Peterson approach for reduction and a separate lateral incision for placement of hardware allows the surgeon optimal visualization.
  - Haidukewych and colleagues[95] showed that the time to surgery was not a risk factor for complications following femoral neck fracture fixation; however, in the case of a Pipkin type III fracture, time to reduction is a known risk factor and thus operative intervention is an orthopedic emergency.[22]
    - The femoral neck fracture must be anatomically reduced, because nonanatomic reduction, especially in varus, leads to a significant increase in failure.[95,101–104]

- After reduction, use of either an SHS with an antirotational screw or 3 to 4 cannulated screws has not been shown to result in differing outcomes, except in Pauwels type III vertical femoral neck fractures, in which an SHS has been shown to decrease the rate of nonunion.[105,106]
- Once the neck fracture is reduced and fixation is obtained, the femoral head may be approached through the methods described earlier.
- In the case of a Pipkin type IV fracture, a femoral head fracture with associated acetabular fracture, the initial approach should be chosen based on the need for fixation of the acetabular fracture.
  - In the case of an acetabular fracture requiring a posterior approach, the surgeon may find that the femoral head fracture is on the anterior aspect of the head.
    - In this case, a surgical dislocation allows optimal visualization of both fracture patterns.
    - Alternatively, dual approaches may be required for intervention of both the femoral head and acetabular fracture. The senior author prefers to position the patient supine and fix the femoral head via a Smith-Peterson approach, followed by a stress examination with fluoroscopy to check posterior hip stability. If unstable, then the patient is repositioned laterally and the posterior injury is addressed via a Kocher approach (Fig. 4).

POSTOPERATIVE CARE

Many clinicians currently allow weight bearing as tolerated with crutches for comfort and to instate posterior or anterior hip precautions for 6 to 8 weeks, depending on the direction of dislocation.[14] The preference of the senior author is to allow touchdown (foot flat) weight bearing with 2-arm support for 6 weeks and to use posterior hip precautions for 3 months. Previously, investigators have recommended bed rest, spica casting, or even temporary traction, despite a stable hip, in an attempt to reduce the rate of avascular necrosis, but at this time the authors are unaware of any studies providing motivation to proceed with more aggressive limitation in activity.[31,32,107]

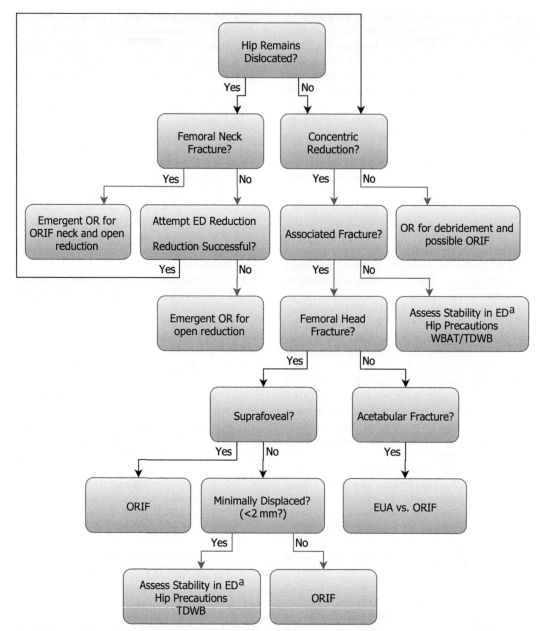

Fig. 4. Our recommended treatment algorithm for hip dislocations. [a] Patients found to have instability should undergo MRI to assess the degree and location of soft tissue injury for possible repair. OR, operating room; ORIF, open reduction with internal fixation; ED, emergency department; EUA, exam under anesthesia; TDWB, touch down weight bearing; WBAT, weight bearing as tolerated.

Open reductions, with or without internal fixation, follow touchdown weight-bearing precautions for 8 to 12 weeks, as well as posterior or anterior hip dislocation precautions for 3 to 6 months. Allowing touchdown (foot flat) weight bearing decreases capsular and fixation strain, although this weight-bearing strategy has not been shown to improve outcomes. Weight bearing is progressed pending radiographic and clinical fracture healing.

COMPLICATIONS AND MANAGEMENT

- Because of modern imaging and standardization of trauma management, modern cohorts do not report on missed or late-diagnosed hip dislocations.[4,5,7,8]
- Surgical infection is not reported as an outlier specific in hip fracture-dislocations; however, several complications and

Table 4
Outcomes based on dislocation type and associated fracture patterns

Study	Dislocation Type	Excellent to Good (%)	Fair to Poor (%)
Upadhyay & Moulton,[4] 1981	Simple	76	24
Armstrong,[35] 1948	Simple	81	19
	Small acetabular fracture	0	100
	Acetabular floor fracture (nonoperative)	0	100
	Femoral head fracture	20	80
Dreinhofer et al,[5] 1994	Simple: anterior	75	25
	Simple: posterior	48	52
Sahin et al,[7] 2003	Simple: posterior	90	10
	Small acetabular fracture	73	27
	Large acetabular fracture	56	44
	Femoral head/neck fracture	0	100
	Simple: anterior	80	20
Thompson & Epstein,[32] 1951	Simple: posterior	67	33
	Large acetabular fracture	32	68
	Comminuted, acetabular floor fracture, or femoral head fracture	10	90

Data from Refs.[4,5,7,32,35]

morbidities affect both closed-treated and open-treated hips:

o Posttraumatic arthritis: overall rates have been reported in 16% to 24% of all hip dislocations,[4,6,7,32,35] and in as many as 89% of those with femoral neck or head fractures.[9] In general, no matter which classification system is used, most clinicians agree that the severity of trauma uniformly increases along the classification scales, and that this severity is the most significant predictor of arthritis.[4,5,10]

o Sciatic nerve palsy: can occur late as result of surgical scarring, or immediately from pressure from the femoral head; iatrogenic injury occurs in up to 12.2% with posterior surgical approach.[108] Time to reduction is directly correlated with the incidence.[22]

o Avascular necrosis: ranges from 6% to 13% for all dislocations[4,7,10]; method of surgical treatment of fracture-dislocation, when indicated, did not affect incidence, but there is direct correlation between time to reduction and avascular necrosis.[10]

o Heterotopic ossification: there is no statistical difference in formation of ectopic bone between patients treated closed versus open; reported rates range from 2.8% to 9%.[7,9,33,35]

OUTCOMES

Long-term results in the literature are often reported on a subjective functional score range of very good to poor, although some investigators do report on radiographic findings or use validated tests such as the Merle d'Aubigne[7,109] functional score. Because several different classifications have been used, as discussed earlier, and several different scoring systems, this article simplifies the reported classification scheme and outcomes where possible into binary results. The studies listed in Table 4 report on long-term outcomes.

Even simple dislocations treated with closed reduction had up to a 52% poor clinical outcome.[4,5] In general, outcome worsened with associated femoral neck or acetabular fractures.

REFERENCES

1. Fairbairn KJ, Mulligan ME, Murphey MD, et al. Gas bubbles in the hip joint on CT: an indication of recent dislocation. AJR Am J Roentgenol 1995;164(4):931–4.

2. Funsten RV, Kinser P, Frankel CJ. Dashboard dislocation of the hip: a report of twenty cases

of traumatic dislocations. J Bone Joint Surg Am 1938;20(1):124–32.

3. Hak DJ, Goulet JA. Severity of injuries associated with traumatic hip dislocation as a result of motor vehicle collisions. J Trauma 1999;47(1):60–3.

4. Upadhyay SS, Moulton A. The long-term results of traumatic posterior dislocation of the hip. J Bone Joint Surg Br 1981;63B(4):548–51.

5. Dreinhofer KE, Schwarzkopf SR, Haas NP, et al. Isolated traumatic dislocation of the hip. Long-term results in 50 patients. J Bone Joint Surg Br 1994;76(1):6–12.

6. Upadhyay SS, Moulton A, Srikrishnamurthy K. An analysis of the late effects of traumatic posterior dislocation of the hip without fractures. J Bone Joint Surg Br 1983;65(2):150–2.

7. Sahin V, Karakas ES, Aksu S, et al. Traumatic dislocation and fracture-dislocation of the hip: a long-term follow-up study. J Trauma 2003;54(3):520–9.

8. Yang RS, Tsuang YH, Hang YS, et al. Traumatic dislocation of the hip. Clin Orthop Relat Res 1991;(265):218–27.

9. Hunter GA. Posterior dislocation and fracture-dislocation of the hip. A review of fifty-seven patients. J Bone Joint Surg Br 1969;51(1):38–44.

10. Stewart MJ, Milford LW. Fracture-dislocation of the hip; an end-result study. J Bone Joint Surg Am 1954;36(A:2):315–42.

11. Frankel VH. Biomechanics of the hip joint. Instr Course Lect 1986;35:3–9.

12. Epstein HC, Wiss DA. Traumatic anterior dislocation of the hip. Orthopedics 1985;8(1):130, 132–4.

13. Chosa E, Tajima N, Nagatsuru Y. Evaluation of acetabular coverage of the femoral head with anteroposterior and false profile radiographs of hip joint. J Orthop Sci 1997;2(6):378–90.

14. Goulet JA. Hip Dislocations. In: Browner BD, Jupiter JB, Krettek C, et al, editors. Skeletal Trauma: Basic Science, Management, and Reconstruction. 5th edition. Philadelphia: Elsevier/Saunders; 2015. p. 1565–95.e4.

15. Stewart KJ, Edmonds-Wilson RH, Brand RA, et al. Spatial distribution of hip capsule structural and material properties. J Biomech 2002;35(11):1491–8.

16. Martin HD, Savage A, Braly BA, et al. The function of the hip capsular ligaments: a quantitative report. Arthroscopy 2008;24(2):188–95.

17. Gautier E, Ganz K, Krügel N, et al. Anatomy of the medial femoral circumflex artery and its surgical implications. J Bone Joint Surg Br 2000;82(5):679–83.

18. Smoll NR. Variations of the piriformis and sciatic nerve with clinical consequence: a review. Clin Anat 2010;23(1):8–17.

19. Nerubay J. Traumatic anterior dislocation of hip joint with vascular damage. Clin Orthop Relat Res 1976;(116):129–32.

20. Eisenberg KS, Sheft DJ, Murray WR. Posterior dislocation of the hip producing lumbosacral nerve-root avulsion. A case report. J Bone Joint Surg Am 1972;54(5):1083–6.

21. Bonnemaison MF, Henderson ED. Traumatic anterior dislocation of the hip with acute common femoral occlusion in a child. J Bone Joint Surg Am 1968;50(4):753–6.

22. Hillyard RF, Fox J. Sciatic nerve injuries associated with traumatic posterior hip dislocations. Am J Emerg Med 2003;21(7):545–8.

23. Gillespie WJ. The incidence and pattern of knee injury associated with dislocation of the hip. J Bone Joint Surg Br 1975;57(3):376–8.

24. Schmidt GL, Sciulli R, Altman GT. Knee injury in patients experiencing a high-energy traumatic ipsilateral hip dislocation. J Bone Joint Surg Am 2005;87(6):1200–4.

25. Tabuenca J, Truan JR. Knee injuries in traumatic hip dislocation. Clin Orthop Relat Res 2000;377(377):78–83.

26. Tornetta P, Kain MSH, Creevy WR. Diagnosis of femoral neck fractures in patients with a femoral shaft fracture. Improvement with a standard protocol. J Bone Joint Surg Am 2007;89(1):39–43.

27. Baird RA, Schobert WE, Pais MJ, et al. Radiographic identification of loose bodies in the traumatized hip joint. Radiology 1982;145(3):661–5.

28. Ebraheim NA, Savolaine ER, Skie MC, et al. Soft-tissue window to enhance visualization of entrapped osteocartilaginous fragments in the hip joint. Orthop Rev 1993;22(9):1017–21.

29. Khanna V, Khanna V, Harris A, et al. Hip arthroscopy: prevalence of intra-articular pathologic findings after traumatic injury of the hip. Arthroscopy 2014;30(3):299–304.

30. Mayer SW, Mayer SW, Stewart JR, et al. MRI as a reliable and accurate method for assessment of posterior hip dislocation in children and adolescents without the risk of radiation exposure. Pediatr Radiol 2015;45(9):1355–62.

31. Clegg TE, Roberts CS, Greene JW, et al. Hip dislocations—epidemiology, treatment, and outcomes. Injury 2010;41(4):329–34.

32. Thompson VP, Epstein HC. Traumatic dislocation of the hip; a survey of two hundred and four cases covering a period of twenty-one years. J Bone Joint Surg Am 1951;33-A(3):746–78. passim.

33. Epstein HC. Traumatic dislocations of the hip. Clin Orthop Relat Res 1973;(92):116–42.

34. Pringle JH, Edwards AH. Traumatic dislocation of the hip joint: an experimental study on the cadaver. Glasgow Med J 1943;21:25–40.

35. Armstrong JR. Traumatic dislocation of the hip joint; review of 101 dislocations. J Bone Joint Surg Br 1948;30B(3):430–45.

36. Marsh JL, Slongo TF, Agel J, et al. Fracture and dislocation classification compendium - 2007: Orthopaedic Trauma Association classification, database and outcomes committee. J Orthop Trauma 2007;21(10 Suppl):S1–133.

37. Bigelow HJ. Luxations of the hip-joint. Boston Med Surg J 1870;82(4):65–7.

38. Allis OH. An inquiry into the difficulties encountered in the reduction of dislocation of the hip. Boston Med Surg J 1896;134(25):625–6.

39. Stimson LA. A treatise on fractures. Philadelphia: H.C. Lea's Son & Co; 1883.

40. Skoff HD. Posterior hip dislocation, a new technique for reduction. Orthop Rev 1986;15(6):405–9.

41. Howard CB. A gentle method of reducing traumatic dislocation of the hip. Injury 1992;23(7): 481–2.

42. Stefanich RJ. Closed reduction of posterior hip dislocation: the Rochester method. Am J Orthop 1999;28(1):64–5.

43. Schafer SJ, Anglen JO. The East Baltimore Lift: a simple and effective method for reduction of posterior hip dislocations. J Orthop Trauma 1999; 13(1):56–7.

44. Ganz R, Gill TJ, Gautier E, et al. Surgical dislocation of the adult hip a technique with full access to the femoral head and acetabulum without the risk of avascular necrosis. J Bone Joint Surg Br 2001;83(8):1119–24.

45. Swiontkowski MF, Thorpe M, Seiler JG, et al. Operative management of displaced femoral head fractures: case-matched comparison of anterior versus posterior approaches for Pipkin I and Pipkin II fractures. J Orthop Trauma 1992;6(4): 437–42.

46. Wylie JD, Abtahi AM, Beckmann JT, et al. Arthroscopic and imaging findings after traumatic hip dislocation in patients younger than 25 years of age. J Hip Preserv Surg 2015;2(3):303–9.

47. Yamamoto Y, Ide T, Ono T, et al. Usefulness of arthroscopic surgery in hip trauma cases. Arthroscopy 2003;19(3):269–73.

48. Matta JM. Operative treatment of acetabular fractures through the ilioinguinal approach. A 10-year perspective. Clin Orthop Relat Res 1994;305(305): 10–9.

49. Mullis BH, Dahners LE. Hip arthroscopy to remove loose bodies after traumatic dislocation. J Orthop Trauma 2006;20(1):22–6.

50. Grimshaw CS, Moed BR. Outcomes of posterior wall fractures of the acetabulum treated nonoperatively after diagnostic screening with dynamic stress examination under anesthesia. J Bone Joint Surg Am 2010;92(17):2792–800.

51. Firoozabadi R, Spitler C, Schlepp C, et al. Determining stability in posterior wall acetabular fractures. J Orthop Trauma 2015;29(10):465–9.

52. Moed BR, Kregor PJ, Reilly MC, et al. Current management of posterior wall fractures of the acetabulum. Instr Course Lect 2015;64:139–59.

53. Grisell M, Moed BR, Bledsoe JG. A biomechanical comparison of trochanteric nail proximal screw configurations in a subtrochanteric fracture model. J Orthop Trauma 2010;24(6):359–63.

54. Davis AT, Moed BR. Can experts in acetabular fracture care determine hip stability after posterior wall fractures using plain radiographs and computed tomography? J Orthop Trauma 2013; 27(10):587–91.

55. Reagan JM, Moed BR. Can computed tomography predict hip stability in posterior wall acetabular fractures? Clin Orthop Relat Res 2011;469(7): 2035–41.

56. Lieberman JR, Altchek DW, Salvati EA. Recurrent dislocation of a hip with a labral lesion: treatment with a modified Bankart-type repair. Case report. J Bone Joint Surg Am 1993;75(10):1524–7.

57. Rashleigh-Belcher HJ, Cannon SR. Recurrent dislocation of the hip with a "Bankart-type" lesion. J Bone Joint Surg Br 1986;68(3):398–9.

58. Birmingham P, Cluett J, Shaffer B. Recurrent posterior dislocation of the hip with a Bankart-type lesion: a case report. Am J Sports Med 2010; 38(2):388–91.

59. Ferguson TA, Patel R, Bhandari M, et al. Fractures of the acetabulum in patients aged 60 years and older: an epidemiological and radiological study. J Bone Joint Surg Br 2010;92(2):250–7.

60. Ferguson SJ, Bryant JT, Ganz R, et al. An in vitro investigation of the acetabular labral seal in hip joint mechanics. J Biomech 2003;36(2):171–8.

61. Ferguson SJ, Bryant JT, Ganz R, et al. The influence of the acetabular labrum on hip joint cartilage consolidation: a poroelastic finite element model. J Biomech 2000;33(8):953–60.

62. Cross MB, Shindle MK, Kelly BT. Arthroscopic anterior and posterior labral repair after traumatic hip dislocation: case report and review of the literature. HSS J 2010;6(2):223–7.

63. Svoboda SJ, Williams DM, Murphy KP. Hip arthroscopy for osteochondral loose body removal after a posterior hip dislocation. Arthroscopy 2003;19(7):777–81.

64. Owens BD, Busconi BD. Arthroscopy for hip dislocation and fracture-dislocation. Am J Orthop 2006;35(12):584–7.

65. Sharma A, Sachdev H, Gomillion M. Abdominal compartment syndrome during hip arthroscopy. Anaesthesia 2009;64(5):567–9.

66. Fowler J, Owens BD. Abdominal compartment syndrome after hip arthroscopy. Arthroscopy 2010;26(1):128–30.

67. Ciemniewska-Gorzela K, Piontek T, Szulc A. Abdominal compartment syndrome – the

prevention and treatment of possible lethal complications following hip arthroscopy: a case report. J Med Case Rep 2014;8(1):368.

68. Keel MJB, Tomagra S, Bonel HM, et al. Clinical results of acetabular fracture management with the pararectus approach. Injury 2014;45(12):1900–7.

69. Canale ST, Manugian AH. Irreducible traumatic dislocations of the hip. J Bone Joint Surg Am 1979;61(1):7–14.

70. Lehtonen R. A study of traumatic dislocations of the hip joint and fractures of the acetabulum. Ann Chir Gynaecol Fenn Suppl 1968;163:1–87.

71. Slätis P, Latvala A. Irreducible traumatic posterior dislocation of the hip. Injury 1974;5(3):188–93.

72. Proctor H. Dislocations of the hip joint (excluding "central" dislocations) and their complications. Injury 1973;5(1):1–12.

73. Brav EA. Traumatic dislocation of the hip. J Bone Joint Surg Am 1962;44(6):1115–34.

74. Miller CH, Gustilo R, Tambornino J. Traumatic hip dislocation. Treatment and results. Minn Med 1971;54(4):253–60.

75. Letournel E. Acetabulum fractures: classification and management. Clin Orthop Relat Res 1980;(151):81–106.

76. Harris AM, Althausen P, Kellam JF, et al. Simultaneous anterior and posterior approaches for complex acetabular fractures. J Orthop Trauma 2008;22(7):494–7.

77. Mayo KA. Open reduction and internal fixation of fractures of the acetabulum. Results in 163 fractures. Clin Orthop Relat Res 1994;305(305):31–7.

78. Baumgaertner MR. Fractures of the posterior wall of the acetabulum. J Am Acad Orthop Surg 1999;7(1):54–65.

79. Keith JE, Brashear HR, Guilford WB. Stability of posterior fracture-dislocations of the hip. Quantitative assessment using computed tomography. J Bone Joint Surg Am 1988;70(5):714.

80. Calkins MS, Zych G, Latta L, et al. Computed tomography evaluation of stability in posterior fracture dislocation of the hip. Clin Orthop Relat Res 1988;227(227):152–63.

81. Siebenrock KA, Tannast M, Bastian JD, et al. Posterior approaches to the acetabulum. Unfallchirurg 2013;116(3):221–6 [in German].

82. Keel MJB, Bastian JD, Büchler L, et al. Surgical dislocation of the hip for a locked traumatic posterior dislocation with associated femoral neck and acetabular fractures. J Bone Joint Surg Br 2010;92(3):442–6.

83. Sagi HC, Bolhofner B. Osteotomy of the anterior superior iliac spine as an adjunct to improve access and visualization through the lateral window. J Orthop Trauma 2015;29(8):e266–9.

84. Letournel E. The treatment of acetabular fractures through the ilioinguinal approach. Clin Orthop Relat Res 1993;(292):62–76.

85. Butterwick D, Papp S, Gofton W, et al. Acetabular fractures in the elderly: evaluation and management. J Bone Joint Surg Am 2015;97(9):758–68.

86. Pagenkopf E, Grose A, Partal G, et al. Acetabular fractures in the elderly: treatment recommendations. HSS J 2006;2(2):161–71.

87. Herscovici D, Lindvall E, Bolhofner B, et al. The combined hip procedure: open reduction internal fixation combined with total hip arthroplasty for the management of acetabular fractures in the elderly. J Orthop Trauma 2010;24(5):291–6.

88. Hougaard K, Thomsen PB. Traumatic posterior fracture-dislocation of the hip with fracture of the femoral head or neck, or both. J Bone Joint Surg Am 1988;70(2):233–9.

89. Epstein HC, Wiss DA, Cozen L. Posterior fracture dislocation of the hip with fractures of the femoral head. Clin Orthop Relat Res 1985;(201):9–17.

90. Roeder LF, DeLee JC. Femoral head fractures associated with posterior hip dislocation. Clin Orthop Relat Res 1980;(147):121–30.

91. Lang-Stevenson A, Getty CJM. The Pipkin fracture-dislocation of the hip. Injury 1987;18(4):264–9.

92. Brumback RJ, Kenzora JE, Levitt LE, et al. Fractures of the femoral head. Hip 1987;181–206.

93. DeLee JC, Evans JA, Thomas J. Anterior dislocation of the hip and associated femoral-head fractures. J Bone Joint Surg Am 1980;62(6):960–4.

94. Greenwald AS, Haynes DW. Weight-bearing areas in the human hip joint. J Bone Joint Surg Br 1972;54(1):157–63.

95. Haidukewych GJ, Rothwell WS, Jacofsky DJ, et al. Operative treatment of femoral neck fractures in patients between the ages of fifteen and fifty years. J Bone Joint Surg Am 2004;86-A(8):1711–6.

96. Marchetti ME, Steinberg GG, Coumas JM. Intermediate-term experience of Pipkin fracture-dislocations of the hip. J Orthop Trauma 1996;10(7):455–61.

97. Stannard JP, Harris HW, Volgas DA, et al. Functional outcome of patients with femoral head fractures associated with hip dislocations. Clin Orthop Relat Res 2000;377(377):44–56.

98. Epstein HC. Posterior fracture-dislocations of the hip; long-term follow-up. J Bone Joint Surg Am 1974;56(6):1103–27.

99. Park K-S, Lee K-B, Na B-R, et al. Clinical and radiographic outcomes of femoral head fractures: excision vs. fixation of fragment in Pipkin type I: what is the optimal choice for femoral head fracture? J Orthop Sci 2015;20(4):702–7.

100. Siebenrock KA, Gautier E, Woo AKH, et al. Surgical dislocation of the femoral head for joint debridement and accurate reduction of fractures

of the acetabulum. J Orthop Trauma 2002;16(8): 543–52.

101. Krischak G, Beck A, Wachter N, et al. Relevance of primary reduction for the clinical outcome of femoral neck fractures treated with cancellous screws. Arch Orthop Trauma Surg 2003;123(8): 404–9.

102. Weinrobe M, Stankewich CJ, Mueller B, et al. Predicting the mechanical outcome of femoral neck fractures fixed with cancellous screws: an in vivo study. J Orthop Trauma 1998;12(1):27–36 [discussion: 36–7].

103. Lowell JD. Results and complications of femoral neck fractures. Clin Orthop Relat Res 1980;(152): 162–72.

104. Bedi A, Karunakar MA, Caron T, et al. Accuracy of reduction of ipsilateral femoral neck and shaft fractures–an analysis of various internal fixation strategies. J Orthop Trauma 2009; 23(4):249–53.

105. Parker MJ, Stockton G. Internal fixation implants for intracapsular proximal femoral fractures in adults. Cochrane Database Syst Rev 2001;(4):CD001467.

106. Liporace F, Gaines R, Collinge C, et al. Results of internal fixation of Pauwels type-3 vertical femoral neck fractures. J Bone Joint Surg Am 2008;90(8): 1654–9.

107. Tornetta P, Mostafavi H. Hip dislocation: current treatment regimens. J Am Acad Orthop Surg 1997;5(1):27–36.

108. Letournel E, Judet R. Fractures of the acetabulum. In: Elson RA, editor. Springer Science & Business Media; 1993. p. 1.

109. d'Aubigné RM, Postel M. Functional results of hip arthroplasty with acrylic prosthesis. J Bone Joint Surg Am 1954;36-A(3):451–75.

Management of Pelvic Ring Injuries in Unstable Patients

Matthew I. Rudloff, MD[a],*, Kostas M. Triantafillou, MD[b]

KEYWORDS

- Unstable pelvic ring injuries • Hemodynamic instability • Polytrauma • Pelvic angiography
- Pelvic packing

KEY POINTS

- Pelvic ring injuries vary in severity and are frequent in the polytrauma patient population.
- A subset of patients presenting with complex pelvic ring injuries and hemodynamic instability require special attention secondary to significant risk of mortality.
- Mortality is bimodal: acutely, from lethal hemorrhage, and late from complications of multiorgan system failure.
- A multidisciplinary approach, and prompt intervention through an algorithmic approach, are necessary to promote survival.
- An understanding of the roles of resuscitation, mechanical pelvic stabilization, angiography, and pelvic packing aid in caring for this subset of extremely injured patients.

ANATOMY

Knowledge of pelvic anatomy is critical to the understanding of pelvic ring injury and treatment. This knowledge allows the surgeon to interpret the readily available bony imaging obtained during the initial trauma assessment, make inferences on pelvic ring stability, temporize life-threatening injuries, anticipate associated injuries, and ultimately definitively stabilize the pelvis to improve long-term functional outcomes.

The function of the pelvis is to transmit weight bearing from the proximal femur to the spine, primarily through the posterior pelvic ring, and to protect the pelvic soft tissue contents. The anterior pelvis, whose injuries are often more easily apparent, plays a secondary role in pelvic stability by functioning primarily as strut. In fact, isolated injuries of the rami or pubic symphysis have little effect on pelvic stability.[1] Because pelvic ring stability is dictated primarily by the posterior ring structures of the sacrum, ilium, and sacroiliac joint, or a combination of these structures, determining stability first requires an understanding of the sacral osteology and the sacroiliac ligamentous complex that connects these entities.

Pelvic osteology is best conceptualized on the inlet and outlet views. On the inlet view, the sacrum is shaped like a reverse keystone (Fig. 1A) to resist the internal rotation vector during weight bearing in conjunction with the transverse oriented fibers of the posterior ligamentous complex and the anterior ring strut. On the outlet view, the sacrum is shaped like a true keystone (Fig. 1B) to resist the medially

Disclosure Statement: Smith & Nephew Orthpaedics, educational consultant; Elsevier, royalties Campbell's Operative Orthopaedics (M.I. Rudloff). K.M. Triantafillou has nothing to disclose.
a Department of Orthopaedic Surgery, Campbell Clinic, University of Tennessee, 1211 Union Avenue, Suite 500, Memphis, TN 38002, USA; b University Orthopedic Surgeons, University of Tennessee Medical Center, 320 Kingston Ct, Knoxville, TN 37919, USA
* Corresponding author.
E-mail address: mrudloff@campbellclinic.com

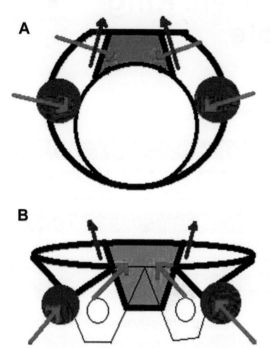

A

B

Fig. 1. (A) Pelvic inlet schematic demonstrating the medial force vector during weight bearing, denoted by the *red arrows*. The shape of the sacrum stabilizes the pelvis from internal rotation deformity. *Blue arrows* indicate the vector of posterior displacement of the hemipelvis in the setting of ligamentous, sacral, or iliac disruption (posterior ring disruption). (B) Pelvic outlet schematic demonstrating cephalomedial force vector during weight bearing, denoted by the *red arrows*. *Blue arrows* denote the vector of cephalad displacement in the setting of posterior ring disruption. The combined vector in the setting of instability is, therefore, posterocephalad displacement.

directed vector during weight bearing in conjunction with the longitudinally oriented fibers of the posterior ligamentous complex. It is easy to see that complete injuries of the sacrum, ligamentous complex, or ilium will result in posterior and cephalad displacement of the hemipelvis.

The posterior sacroiliac ligamentous complex is a collective term inclusive of the multiple ligaments that confer stability to the sacroiliac joints, connecting the ilium to the sacrum. Of these, the interosseous sacroiliac ligaments are the strongest and run transversely from the posterior superior and inferior spine of the ilium to the posterior sacrum. Posteriorly, the short and long posterior sacroiliac ligaments, collectively the posterior sacroiliac ligaments, run obliquely and longitudinally. The anterior sacroiliac ligaments pass transversely from the anterior sacrum to the anterior edge of the ilium (Fig. 2). The sacrotuberous ligament is confluent with the posterior sacroiliac ligament and runs longitudinally to the ischial tuberosity (Fig. 3) and forms the border of the greater sciatic notch along with the weight-bearing arch of the ilium. Another longitudinally oriented ligament is the sacrospinous ligament (see Fig. 3), which, as its name suggests, connects the sacrum to the iliac spine and forms the border of the lesser sciatic notch along with the ilium and sacrotuberous ligament. Finally, the iliolumbar ligament connects the L5 transverse process to the iliac crest (see Fig. 3).

The posterior ligaments contribute most to resisting forces across the sacroiliac joint and are known collectively as the posterior tension band. The transversely oriented fibers primarily resist rotational forces, whereas the longitudinally oriented ligaments are the primary restraint against vertical shear forces. The combination and degree of injuries to these ligaments, along with disruption to the sacrum or ilium, explains the wide spectrum of stability seen in pelvic ring injuries.

Knowledge of structures at risk for injury after a pelvic ring injury is essential because it directs the physical examination for life-threatening injuries and provides clues to pelvic stability for selecting provisional or definitive fixation.

Peripheral nerve deficit may occur with wide displacement of the hemipelvis and indicate

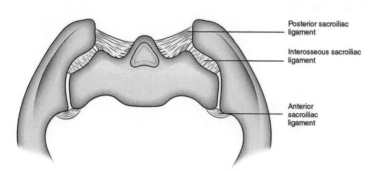

Posterior sacroiliac ligament

Interosseous sacroiliac ligament

Anterior sacroiliac ligament

Fig. 2. The primary sacroiliac ligaments as demonstrated on a schematic pelvic inlet diagram. The posterior ligaments function similarly to a suspension bridge, resisting internal rotation deformity, whereas the anterior sacroiliac ligaments primarily restrain against external rotation forces. The interosseous sacroiliac ligaments, centered between them, are the strongest in the pelvis.

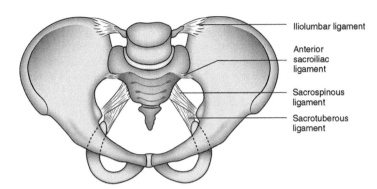

Fig. 3. Schematic anteroposterior pelvis with the stabilizing ligaments of the pelvic ring. Sacrotuberous, sacrospinous, and anterior sacroiliac ligaments provide resistance to external rotation, whereas longitudinal fibers within these ligaments in conjunction with the posterior ligamentous complex (not shown) and the iliolumbar ligaments providing stability against vertical displacement.

the possibility of complete hemipelvis instability. The lumbosacral plexus (**Fig. 4**) is derived from the anterior rami of the T12 to S4 nerve roots and courses anteriorly to the sacroiliac joint. The L4, L5, S1, and S2 nerve roots are of surgical importance because they may be injured with aberrant placement of sacroiliac screws during percutaneous fixation with sacroiliac screws or with open reduction and internal fixation of the sacroiliac joint.

Death from hemorrhage is the primary concern during the management of pelvic injuries in the unstable patient. Although blood loss is most commonly due to disruption of the pelvic venous plexus, injuries to the arteries of the pelvis can occur in isolation or combination (see **Fig. 6**). The median sacral artery, superior rectal, and iliac artery are the main arteries of the pelvis. However, it is injury to the internal iliac artery that most commonly results in early mortality.

Urethral tears, especially in males, are a common cause of comorbidity after pelvic trauma. Disruption of the sacrotuberous and sacrospinous ligaments during pelvic displacement may result in tension and injury to the pelvic floor. The urethra pierces the pelvic floor and is particularly vulnerable at this level, which may result in injury requiring repair.

CLINICAL ASSESSMENT

The clinical assessment of the patient is of utmost importance because the radiographic assessment most often underestimates the degree of pelvic instability seen at the time of injury owing to hemipelvis recoil, placement of a pelvic binder, and the reducing effect of the concave computed tomography (CT) table. The initial physical examination, as always, begins with a general assessment of the multiply injured patient as directed by the principles of Advanced Trauma Life Support (ATLS) guidelines. For the purposes of this review, discussion is limited to the examination of pelvic ring injuries in the polytrauma patient. Assessment begins with a history that will alert the examiner to potentially life-threatening injuries of the pelvis.

The mechanism of injury provides an overall assessment of the energy imparted to the patient, with high-energy mechanisms such as motor vehicle accidents, falls from considerable height, and industrial accidents resulting in the greatest degree of instability patterns. Determining the direction of force may help with assessing injury patterns. However, descriptions of the direction of force may confound the assessment because high-energy mechanisms

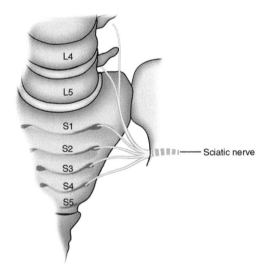

L4

L5

S1

S2

S3

S4

S5

Sciatic nerve

Fig. 4. The lumbosacral plexus is associated intimately with the posterior ring, and is therefore at risk with posterior ring disruption. Neurologic deficits may occur with massive displacement of the pelvic ring at the time of injury, and are highly suggestive of pelvic ring instability despite unimpressive initial radiographs.

often result in multiple force vectors with resulting combined instability patterns that may be overlooked. Also overlooked is the impact of the age of the patient. Pelvic ring injuries in the young require substantially high energy, and can call into question a seemingly low-energy injury mechanism. The elderly require a high index of suspicion, because although most pelvic ring injuries are due to bony insufficiency, high-energy pelvic injuries in the elderly have extremely high mortality.[2] Medical history is also important, because it provides a risk assessment, particularly in patients with coagulopathy owing to disease or medication.

The examination begins with an interpretation of vital signs. Pelvic fractures are responsible for approximately 15% of deaths in the polytrauma population,[3] of which acute hemorrhage is the most common etiology. Therefore, in the setting of the unstable patient, attention is turned to identify causes of hemorrhage. A systolic blood pressure of less than 104 mm Hg and need for transfusion in the trauma bay are independent predictors of pelvic fracture related arterial bleeding.[4] The ATLS workup should exclude external, thoracic, and abdominal causes of hemorrhage. The presence of hemodynamic instability with a concomitant anteroposterior (AP) radiograph showing a displaced pelvic ring injury should prompt immediate intervention. It should be noted that a femur fracture, in isolation, should not cause hemodynamic instability, and should not draw attention from the pelvic ring injury.

The examination continues with inspection and palpation of the perineum, rectum, and vagina for open fractures, because open pelvic fractures, along with vascular injury, carry a 50% incidence of mortality.[5] Contusions should be noted and provide clues toward instability patterns and alert the surgeon to Morel–Lavalle lesions. The urethra, especially in males, should be inspected for blood, because this finding may indicate a urogenital injury. Leg length discrepancy and rotation should also be examined and documented.

The pelvis should then be stressed with internal and externally directed force to feel for instability. This examination should be performed only once, because repeated examination may result in the loss of tamponade and hemodynamic instability in the presence of an unstable ring injury. Often, instability in the pelvis can be inferred from the initial pelvic radiograph. In this situation, "stress" evaluation of the pelvis may be unnecessary potentially avoiding disruption of early clot formation.

Neurologic examination is critical. A careful neurologic examination may reveal peripheral nerve deficiency caused by large displacement of the pelvis at the time of injury. In the absence of a known cause, this finding almost invariably indicates an unstable pelvic ring injury.

RADIOGRAPHIC ASSESSMENT

The AP pelvis radiograph is part of the ATLS evaluation and provides the initial information needed to determine whether hemodynamic instability may be owing to a pelvic ring disruption. Significant pubic symphysis diastasis with resultant external rotation of the hemipelvis increases the pelvic volume and provides a large space for hemorrhage. Gross vertical displacement may also be seen, indicating pelvic instability. Other subtle signs of gross instability include ischial spine or sacral avulsion fractures (indicating sacrotuberous or sacrospinous ligament incompetence), or a fracture of the L5 transverse process, where the iliolumbar ligament attaches. Posterior ring instability can occur through either failure of the sacroiliac ligaments leading to a widened sacroiliac joint, through complete fracture through the sacrum at the S1 and S2 vertebral levels, or through fracture of the ilium. Although specific, the AP radiograph alone is not sensitive and requires inlet and outlet views to better demonstrate posterior and cephalad displacement, respectively.

CT scan of the chest, abdomen, and pelvis is performed routinely in the polytrauma patient after the primary and secondary surveys. The CT scan better characterizes the often difficult to visualize posterior pelvic ring injury compared with radiographs. Instability is characterized by complete fractures of the sacrum or ilium, or widening of the sacroiliac joint, and is most useful for preoperative planning of definitive fracture management. However, it should be noted that the standard pelvic radiographs offer a better assessment of gross pelvic rotation and posterior or cephalad displacement for determining the need for pelvic binder and/or traction in the acute setting.

CLASSIFICATION

Classifications are useful in that they simplify the spectrum of complex injury patterns, enhance provider communication, predict prognosis and associated injuries, and help guide decision making. The Tile classification will be described and correlated with the Young–Burgess classification to draw on the strengths of both. The Tile classification is categorized into type A, or stable pelvic ring injury; type B, or partially stable pelvic ring injury; and type C, or completely unstable pelvic ring injury (Fig. 5).

In type A injuries, the integrity of the posterior pelvic ring, and therefore the weight-bearing arch of the pelvis, remains intact. Type A injuries include avulsion fractures and iliac wing or isolated anterior ring injuries owing to a direct blow. These injuries do not cause hemodynamic instability.

Type B injuries, or partially unstable pelvic ring injuries, comprise a wide spectrum of injury patterns that may or may not contribute to hemodynamic instability. Type B injuries include AP compression injuries (Young–Burgess anteroposterior compression [APC] I and APC 2), which result in an "open book" deformity in which the hemipelvis is unstable in external rotation. In this injury, the pubis symphysis, and anterior sacroiliac and pelvic floor ligaments may be attenuated or disrupted, but the posterior sacroiliac ligaments remain intact. Differentiating the degree of instability requires examination if gross external rotation is not present. A rotationally unstable hemipelvis in external rotation may result in tension and injury to the pelvic vasculature, leading to hemodynamic instability if left untreated in the acute setting.

Type B injuries also include lateral compression injuries (Young–Burgess lateral compression [LC] 1 and LC 2), in which the anterior pelvic "strut" fails in internal rotation, leading to various degrees of posterior ring injury. However, the integrity of the pelvic floor and sacrospinous and sacrotuberous ligaments remains intact. These injuries are not often implicated in hemodynamic instability because shortening, rather than tension, occurs across the pelvic vascular structures, but do have a high association with mortality from head injuries. Last, type B injuries also include the "windswept pelvis," in which lateral compression of 1 hemipelvis occurs, causing an external rotation moment, and "open book" injury to the contralateral pelvis.

Type C injuries, or complete pelvic instability, occur with complete displacement of the sacrum, ilium, or complete rupture of the sacroiliac ligamentous complex. Type C injuries include the Young–Burgess APC III, vertical shear, and many combined injury patterns. These injuries are associated most often with hemodynamic instability, large transfusion requirement on presentation, and death.[6]

INITIAL MANAGEMENT

The trauma evaluation is a multidisciplinary approach and should be performed in a systematic

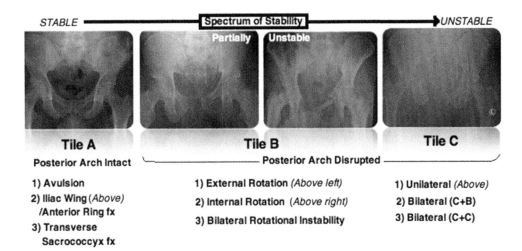

Fig. 5. Tile classification. Representative anteroposterior pelvis radiographs demonstrate the continuous spectrum but pattern variability of posterior ring disruption. Tile A injuries do not involve the weight bearing arch, and suggest an extrapelvic etiology of hemodynamic instability, if present. A rotational injury without cephalad displacement indicates a partially stable posterior ring (tile B), which may or may not be causative of hemodynamic instability. External rotation injury patterns within this group have a higher likelihood for intrapelvic hemorrhage and should be addressed acutely. Concomitant cephalad and/or wide posterior displacement of the hemipelvis suggests complete posterior ring injury (tile C), and requires high suspicion for pelvic etiology of hemodynamic instability. These patterns require both axial traction and internal rotation devices (binders) in the acute setting.

fashion. The focus is on initial management of the unstable patient. The first step in evaluating a patient with an injury to the pelvic ring, is obtaining a history, including an understanding of the mechanism of injury. The history may not be obtainable from the patient in some circumstances, and reports from the first responders may lend insight into the injury. The mechanism of injury raises the index of suspicion for concomitant system injuries. ATLS protocols are instituted, following the *ABCDE*s for methodical appraisal of the injuries:

- Airway,
- Breathing,
- Circulation,
- Disability, and
- Exposure.

Higher energy mechanisms rarely cause pelvic ring disruptions in isolation. In addition to multisystem injuries, 60% to 80% of patients with high-energy pelvic ring disruptions will also have another musculoskeletal injury. Twelve percent of patients will have associated urogenital injuries, and 8% of patients will have lumbosacral plexus injuries[7] (Fig. 6).

Airway stabilization, breathing support, and circulatory problems are the priorities during the initial survey. The etiology of hypotension should be aggressively sought, and acute blood loss can be estimated based on physiologic parameters, and may guide resuscitation requirements. During the exposure portion of the evaluation, careful evaluation may reveal the presence of ecchymosis, soft tissue fullness, open wounds or lacerations, limb length

discrepancies, and musculoskeletal instability. Urogenital and rectal examinations are mandatory. Although stress evaluation of the pelvis has been advocated, it has been shown to have poor sensitivity (59%) and specificity (71%).[8] It is important to realize that the pelvic ring injury may only be 1 component of a constellation of injuries accounting for hemodynamic instability.

Initial imaging aids in identifying the potential sources of hemorrhage. Chest radiographs, and more recently ultrasound imaging, can identify and rule out hemopneumothoraces. Although the clinical abdominal examination may seem benign in an obtunded patient, the use of abdominal ultrasound can accurately recognize intraabdominal bleeding. The Focused Assessment with Sonography in Trauma (FAST) examination can provide rapid information in identifying location of hemorrhage, simultaneously during other resuscitative measures, and without the time delay of CT scan. The AP pelvic radiograph can demonstrate quickly a gross deformity or instability of the pelvic ring, and the orthopedic surgeon should also recognize injury patterns that have the potential for instability, and whether mechanical stabilization of the pelvis is needed.

In the absence of other major sources of bleeding, the pelvic ring injury should be addressed quickly. The ultimate goal is to provide stability to the pelvis to decrease the pelvic volume and decrease ongoing pelvic hemorrhage. This is most applicable to APC injuries, and generally LC injury patterns will not benefit, and has the potential for exaggerating deformity. Several modalities are available to provide emergent stabilization of the injured pelvis. These include circumferential sheets, commercially available pelvic binders, military antishock trousers, C-clamps, and lower extremity taping with each having advantages and disadvantages. Tile C injuries may also benefit from skeletal traction in the acute setting to control proximal and posterior displacement.

Military antishock trousers were used historically as an initial means of addressing hypotension associated with acute blood loss; however, they were not found to decrease mortality, duration of hospitalization, or duration of intensive care stay, and have largely been replaced by simpler methods.[9] A folded sheet can provide compression to the injured pelvis in a simple, noninvasive, and cost-effective manner.[10] Alternatively, commercially available pelvic binders are readily available in most trauma centers. In either circumstance, the ideal position is located

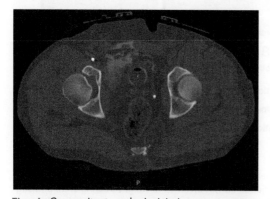

Fig. 6. Concomitant urologic injuries are common. This axial computed tomography cystogram image demonstrates contrast extravasation consistent with an extraperitoneal bladder rupture. Appropriate consultation is necessary particularly when planning definitive anterior fixation.

over the greater trochanters. This location requires the least tension required for reduction of the pelvis.[11] Simple in design and application, one still must be cognizant of the potential soft tissue implications of prolonged wear. Nonetheless, pelvic binders have been reported to decrease transfusion requirements, length of hospitalization, and mortality in patients with APC injuries[12] (Fig. 7).

External fixation is another modality that can provide stability to the injured pelvis. This can be performed with an anterior uniplanar construct, or with a pelvic C-clamp. Anterior pelvic external fixation can effectively reduce a rotationally unstable injury, and has been shown to increase the retroperitoneal pressures potentially aiding in tamponade.[13] An anterior frame alone, however, may be less effective in controlling a significantly displaced posterior ring injury. The pelvic C-clamp can better control posterior injuries owing to its ability for placement on the posterior ilium, but is technically more difficult and time consuming to position. These devices are usually best applied in an operating room, with fluoroscopy, which requires valuable time during the initial evaluation and resuscitation phase. Therefore, circumferential pelvic compression should be considered the initial treatment for a rotationally unstable pelvis in the setting of hemodynamic instability on presentation given the rapidity and ease with which it can be applied in the trauma bay. Conversion to more definitive stabilization, even if temporary, can then occur after a successful resuscitation.

RESUSCITATION

During the initial evaluation to establish sites of hemorrhage and to control them, fluid resuscitation is performed concomitantly to address hypotension. Controversy exists regarding the "ideal" formula for fluid resuscitation. High-volume crystalloid infusions after trauma have been linked with abdominal compartment syndrome, acute respiratory distress syndrome, multiple organ failure, and coagulation disturbances.[14–16] Therefore, a more conservative approach to crystalloid utilization has occurred, and a damage control resuscitation focus has emerged. Initial therapy begins with 2 L of crystalloid before component therapy, or massive transfusion protocols are instituted to those patients unresponsive to this first step.

Trauma-induced coagulopathy can predict transfusion need and mortality risk, and is

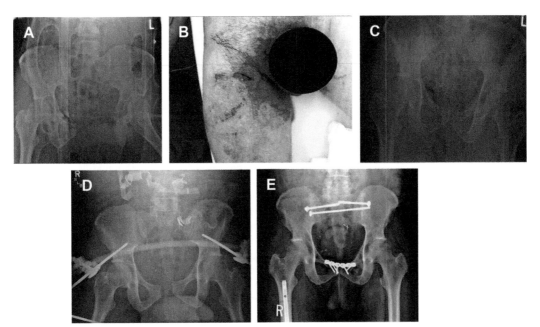

Fig. 7. (A) Initial trauma anteroposterior pelvic radiograph in a 46-year-old man after a high-speed motorcycle crash. (B) The injury was open through a soft tissue degloving injury to the right groin. (C) After pelvic binder placement in the trauma bay. Note the significant reduction that can be achieved by this simple tactic. (D) After laparotomy, the binder was converted to a low anterior external fixator at the time of debridement and irrigation. (E) Definitive stabilization can then occur in a delayed fashion.

potentiated by acidosis, and hypothermia[17] Hemodilution, in the absence of acidosis and hypothermia, has been found to have little effect on coagulation after trauma.[18] Massive transfusion protocols continue to evolve as the pathophysiology for trauma-induced coagulopathy advances.[19] Traditionally, trauma-induced coagulopathy has been postulated to be the result of depleted, dysfunctional, and diluted coagulation factors; however, this phenomenon is a much more complex disruption of the delicate balance between procoagulants, anticoagulants, platelets, endothelium, and fibrinolysis.[20]

The optimal transfusion ratio during resuscitation is still under investigation. In those patients requiring massive transfusions for resuscitation, mortality was decreased with a plasma:red blood cell (RBC) ratio of >1:2, a platelet:RBC ratio of 1:1, and a cryoprecipitate:RBC ratio of 1:1.[21–25] However, there is concern regarding "survivor bias" in the massive transfusion literature, in that early deaths were frequently in the low ratio groups because the plasma administration was started after the RBC infusion.[26] In a prospective study, the PROMMTT Study Group demonstrated increased plasma:RBC and platelet:RBC ratios as independent predictors for decreased 6-hour mortality in patients at risk for hemorrhagic death. Furthermore, those with plasma:RBC and platelet:RBC ratios of less than 1:2 were 3 to 4 times more likely to die when compared with those with ratios of 1:1 or higher.[27]

The strategy of damage control resuscitation is an extension of the principles of damage control surgery for the care of critically injured patients. It focuses on early blood product administration, addressing ongoing hemorrhage, and restoration of physiologic parameters, particularly avoiding the lethal triad of coagulopathy, acidosis, and hypothermia.

DAMAGE CONTROL RESUSCITATION

- Rapid control of hemorrhage.
- Early use of blood products (RBCs, plasma, and platelets in 1:1:1 ratio).
- Avoid excessive crystalloid use.
- Prevention of hypothermia and acidosis.
- Permissive hypotension.

When using damage control resuscitation, patients are treated empirically for trauma-induced coagulopathy with blood components in fixed ratios. As the resuscitation progresses, point-of-care coagulation testing can be used to identify specific coagulation deficiencies to theoretically allow a more focused correction. Goal-directed damage control resuscitation has been reported to decrease transfusions and improve outcomes.[28] However, a subsequent systematic review concluded that the effect of point-of-care testing on blood product transfusion, mortality, and outcomes remain unproven.[29]

Recombinant factor VIIa was previously used in an off-label fashion for additional bleeding control in those requiring massive transfusion protocols. Morse and colleagues[30] demonstrated decreased 24-hour mortality in patients receiving greater than 30 units of packed RBCs; however, this initial decrease was not maintained at 30 days after injury. Risks include potentiating a thromboembolic state.

Tranexamic acid has shown a lessened need for transfusion in elective surgery.[31] A large randomized placebo-controlled trial of trauma patients revealed mortality reduction of 1.5% in the tranexamic acid group (14.5% vs 16.0%) at 28 days and those from hemorrhage from 5.7% to 4.9%. In a smaller subset of patients presenting with a systolic blood pressure of less than 75 mm Hg, 28-day mortality in the tranexamic acid group was 30.6% versus 35.1% for placebo.[32] An increase in mortality was noted with administration more than 3 hours from injury. The exact role of these agents as adjuvant treatments during damage control resuscitation using massive transfusion protocols is yet to be determined.

ROLE OF ANGIOGRAPHY

After initial mechanical stabilization of the injured pelvis and appropriate fluid resuscitation efforts, patients in whom suspected ongoing bleeding is occurring, should be considered for angiography. In many centers in the United States, angiography is the first-line treatment of choice. The timing of this intervention can vary depending on the clinical scenario and institutional factors. Burgess and colleagues[33] reported on a series of 162 patients with high-energy pelvic ring injuries; 7.0% underwent angiography, the majority requiring embolization were APC and vertical shear patterns of injury. In their series of 325 patients, Starr and colleagues[34] reported 10% undergoing arteriography, and found that age (>60 years) and Revised Trauma Score to be predictive of the need for this modality. Systolic blood pressure on arrival, shock on arrival, and base deficit were not associated with the use of pelvic angiography. In another series, Eastridge and colleagues[35] noted that in patients with stable pelvic injuries (LC 1, APC 1) who had ongoing hemorrhage, an abdominal source was found in 85%. In contrast, in those with unstable ring injuries, a pelvic source was identified in 59%, concluding that angiography should be considered before laparotomy. The timing of angiography in the sequence of resuscitation remains debatable.

Although angiography is effective in treating an arterial source, it is ineffective in addressing hemorrhage from venous sources or fracture sites. Venous bleeding is accountable in approximately 85% of patients with hemorrhage attributed to the pelvis. Angiography requires additional resources and specialty personnel to be available, is necessary during a critical time in the resuscitation process, and may not be targeting the most common etiology. Furthermore, it may delay treatment of concomitant injuries. Hou and colleagues[36] reported on their series of 48 patients with hemodynamically unstable pelvic injuries. After ATLS protocol, 12 patients underwent angiography with embolization, with mean time to the procedure 3 hours 55 minutes

(range, 2–19 hours), and an overall mortality rate of 41.7%. Others have reported that embolization within 3 hours of arrival had greater survival rates, with range 50 minutes to 19 hours.[37] Balogh and colleagues[38] reported on the effectiveness of following institutional practice guidelines, including angiography performed within 90 minutes of admission, revealing a decrease in mortality rates.

Angiography is an effective tool in the management of the hemodynamically unstable pelvis when an arterial source is suspected (Fig. 8). However, angiography can be resource and personnel dependent. It has potential ischemic risks, particularly in the setting of nonspecific applications. Resulting ischemia can compromise definitive surgical approaches. Furthermore, not all arterial bleeding may be noted on initial angiography secondary to vasospasm (see Fig. 8). However, in most centers it is typically indicated for those patients experiencing ongoing hemorrhage despite pelvic sheet, binder, or external fixation, and no other identified bleeding source. Contrast-enhanced CT scan can identify arterial bleeding that could

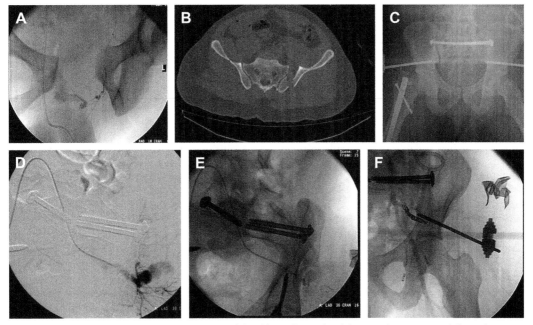

Fig. 8. (A) Pelvic angiography addressing anterior bleed from the pudendal artery that was noted through an open perineal wound. (B) Computed tomography scan demonstrating the extent of the posterior ring injury. (C) Stabilization of the pelvis, after debridement and irrigation, with external fixation, and posterior percutaneous fixation. External fixation was used definitively secondary to the extent of perineal soft tissue injury. (D, E) The patient developed delayed gluteal compartment syndrome secondary to a bleeding superior gluteal pseudoaneurysm at the level of his sacroiliac fracture dislocation. No extravasation was noted at initial angiography from this location. (F) Pseudoaneurysm treated with angioembolization, after evacuation of hematoma. The ideal indication for angiography is when a specific arterial source is suspected.

benefit from angiography; however, in the unstable patient CT scanning may be ill-advised until circulatory control is achieved.

ROLE OF PELVIC PACKING

An alternative to angiography, pelvic packing can provide a simple but effective modality for hemorrhage control. Frequently reported in Europe, this technique has not been widely used in North America. Pelvic packing is effective against venous sources and smaller arterial bleeds, and provides the opportunity for direct ligation. Direct ligation risks iatrogenic neural injury secondary to the proximity of the lumbosacral plexus, and is usually avoided unless a major visualized source is noted. Hemostasis is typically obtained by tamponade with surgical packing of the presacral and paravesical regions. Pelvic packing is best accomplished in combination with mechanical stabilization of the pelvis, with either external fixation or pelvic C-clamp application, depending on the osseous injury pattern.

First described in Hannover, Germany, direct hemostatic control with packing for tamponade has gained in popularity in Europe.[39] Ertel and colleagues[40] demonstrated that acute application of a pelvic C-clamp and subsequent pelvic packing for hemorrhage without angiography and embolization was successful, and suggested serial lactate levels to assess severity of hemorrhage. The technique has been refined, and recently in the United States, Cothren and colleagues[41] reported on their series of pelvic injuries presenting with hemodynamic instability, following an institutional protocol. Twenty-eight consecutive patients underwent external fixation and preperitoneal pelvic packing. This technique was performed through an 8 cm midline vertical incision, and 6 to 7 laparotomy pads were placed rapidly, usually 3 on either side of the bladder, and 1 anteriorly if space required. The postprocedure transfusion requirements were significantly less. The first 4 patients underwent routine angiography, with 1 requiring embolization. Four patients underwent subsequent angiography with embolization for concerns of persistent hemorrhage. No deaths resulted from acute blood loss.

In their follow-up study, the authors evaluated 75 consecutive patients under the same institutional algorithm.[42] After preperitoneal pelvic packing/external fixation, 10 patients (13%) underwent angioembolization. Again, significantly less blood product administration was necessary in the first 24-hour postoperative period. Fifteen patients (20%) required repeat packing upon reinspection, with a mean time for packing removal of 2 days (range, 1–7). This study further demonstrated no deaths owing to acute blood loss, and with an overall mortality rate of 21%, which was significantly lower than previous mortality rates. The authors concluded that this protocol was effective in controlling hemodynamically unstable pelvic injuries, citing that packing directly addressed the most common cause of hemorrhage and decreased the need for transfusion, an independent risk factor for mortality.[43] The authors reserved angiography as an adjuvant treatment for the subset of patients with ongoing bleeding.

Pelvic packing is not without disadvantages. Comparatively, pelvic packing is more invasive than angiography and infectious complications can occur. Cothren and colleagues[42] reported a 15% pelvic space infection rate. Infection was noted in 6 patients with open fractures or perineal degloving soft tissue injuries, 3 patients with bladder disruptions, and 5 patients without bowel or bladder pathology. Pelvic space infections were more common in those requiring repeat packing versus single packing (47% vs 6%), thus questioning the timing or role of repacking.

TIMING OF DEFINITIVE FIXATION

The timing of definitive fixation begins with a critical appraisal of the resuscitation progress. Successful resuscitation from hemorrhagic shock is gauged by a combination of physiologic and laboratory parameters. Common parameters include decreased heart rate, normalized blood pressure, and satisfactory urine production (30 mL/h). Despite normal parameters, insufficient end tissue oxygenation can still occur, and therefore these parameters should not be relied upon solely.

Serum lactate can serve as a diagnostic marker in treatment of hemorrhagic shock; it is a byproduct of anaerobic glycolysis and indirectly represents tissue hypoperfusion. Vincent and colleagues[44] demonstrated that serial lactate measurements can provide valuable information early in the resuscitation regarding responsiveness. Abramson and colleagues[45] reported data regarding lactate clearance and correlation with survival in multitrauma. When lactate levels normalized (<2 mmol/L) within 24 hours, all patients in their series survived. However, survival decreased to 77.8% and 13.6% when lactate levels corrected within 48 hours and greater than 48 hours, respectively.

Elevated lactate levels, beyond 24 hours, has been linked to posttraumatic organ failure, and initial lactate levels were higher in nonsurvivors of trauma.[46]

In parallel, base deficit has been shown to be predictive of mortality with hemorrhagic shock secondary to trauma.[47] Davis and colleagues[48] defined three degrees of base deficit, mild (−3 to −5 mEq/L), moderate (−6 to −9 mEq/L) and severe (<−10 mEq/L), correlating with initial 24-hour transfusions and risk for organ failure and mortality. In a separate study, the same group identified base deficit as superior to pH from arterial blood gas sampling for prediction of death.[49]

Although both lactate and base deficit have diagnostic value, the do not necessarily correlate with each other.[50] Paladino and colleagues[51] evaluated the use of these two parameters (lactate, >2.2 mmol/L; base deficit, <−2.0 mEq), in conjunction with abnormal vital signs (heart rate >100 bpm or systolic blood pressure <90 mm Hg) for recognizing major traumatic injuries, which increased the sensitivity for major injury from 40.9% to 76.4%.

Definitive management of the injured pelvis should only be undertaken when resuscitation is deemed complete. This implies normalization of not only physiologic parameters, but also objective data with serial monitoring of lactate and base deficit.

TREATMENT ALGORITHM

Although debate continues regarding the optimal role and timing for certain treatment modalities, particularly angiography and pelvic packing, the goals of treatment are clear. Care of the critically injured hypotensive patients with pelvic ring injuries centers around expeditious principle-based, multidisciplinary treatment to quickly stop potentially lethal hemorrhage, stabilize the pelvis, and administer appropriate resuscitation to increase survivability.

Immediately upon arrival, or in prehospital care, patient resuscitation should begin with conservative crystalloid infusion (2 L). If the patient improves, the standard trauma imaging follows. Those who fail to respond physiologically should receive component blood product therapy as part of a massive transfusion protocol in a 1:1:1 ratio. Concomitantly, the mechanically unstable pelvis must be stabilized upon diagnosis in the trauma bay, with a pelvis sheet or binder being the easiest. Peripheral sites of hemorrhage should be controlled with packing and or splinted as dictated. If an intraabdominal source of bleeding is identified via FAST or

diagnostic peritoneal lavage, then the patient is transported to the operating suite for exploratory laparotomy. Consideration should be given to application of more rigid pelvic stabilization with external fixation and possibly pelvic packing. Angiography with selective embolization can still provide benefit for those with concerns for ongoing bleeding.

Controversy, however, exists when no other sources of bleeding are identified (thorax or abdomen), and the patient remains hypotensive despite appropriate fluid management. The pelvis must be presumed to be the source. Many centers favor angiography as the first-line treatment in this circumstance, despite the relatively small percentage of arterial injuries accounting for this clinical scenario. In contrast, European and limited US centers have advocated external fixation with pelvic packing as the first line treatment, reserving angiography for those with persistent blood loss. Both angiography, and pelvic packing should be considered tools in the armamentarium of care and should be viewed as complimentary, because each targets specific but separate bleeding sources. The roles of each should be appreciated by the orthopedic surgeon charged with caring for this demanding injury subset.

REFERENCES

1. Tile M, Helfet DL, Kellam JF, et al. Fractures of the pelvis and acetabulum. 3rd edition. Philadelphia: Lippincott, Williams & Wilkins; 2003. p. 32.
2. Keller J, Sciadini MF, Sinclair E, et al. Geriatric trauma: demographics, injuries, and mortality. J Orthop Trauma 2012;26(9):e161–5.
3. Chong K, DeCoster T, Osler T, et al. Pelvic fractures and mortality. Iowa Orthop J 1997;17:110.
4. Toth L, King KL, McGrath B, et al. Factors associated with pelvic fracture-related arterial bleeding during trauma resuscitation: a prospective clinical study. J Orthop Trauma 2014;28(9):489–95.
5. Richardson JD, Harty J, Amin M, et al. Open pelvic fractures. J Trauma 1982;22(7):533–8.
6. Ruatti S, Guillot S, Brun J, et al. Which pelvic ring fractures are potentially lethal? Injury 2015;46(6): 1059–63.
7. McMurtry R, Walton D, Dickinson D, et al. Pelvic disruption in the polytraumatized patient: a management protocol. Clin Orthop Relat Res 1980;(151):22–30.
8. Grant PT. The diagnosis of pelvic fractures by "springing". Arch Emerg Med 1990;7:178–82.
9. Dickinson K, Roberts I. Medical anti-shock trousers (pneumatic anti-shock garments) for circulatory

10. Routt ML Jr, Falicov A, Woodhouse E, et al. Circumferential pelvic antishock sheeting: a temporary resuscitation aid. J Orthop Trauma 2002;16(1):45–8.

11. Bottland M, Krieg JC, Mohr M, et al. Emergent management of pelvic ring fractures with use of circumferential compression. J Bone Joint Surg Am 2002;84-A(Suppl 2):43–7.

12. Croce MA, Magnotti LJ, Savage SA, et al. Emergent pelvic fixation in patients with exsanguinating pelvic fractures. J Am Coll Surg 2007;204:935–42.

13. Grimm MR, Vrahas MS, Thomas KA. Pressure-volume characteristics of the intact and disrupted pelvic retroperitoneum. J Trauma 1998;44(3):454–9.

14. Moore FA, McKinley BA, Moore EE. The next generation in shock resuscitation. Lancet 2004;363:1988–96.

15. Cotton BA, Guy JS, Morris JA Jr, et al. The cellular, metabolic and systemic consequences of aggressive fluid resuscitation strategies. Shock 2006;26(2):115–21.

16. Wideemann HP, Wheeler AP, Bernard GR, et al. Comparison of two fluid-management strategies in acute lung injury. N Engl J Med 2006;354:2564–75.

17. Eddy VA, Morris JA Jr, Cullinane DC. Hypothermia coagulopathy, and acidosis. Surg Clin North Am 2000;80:845–54.

18. Wohlauer MV, Moore EE, Droz NM, et al. Hemodilution is not critical in the pathogenesis of the acute coagulopathy of trauma. J Surg Res 2012;173:26–30.

19. Pohlman T, Walsh M, Aversa J, et al. Damage control resuscitation. Blood Rev 2015;29(4):251–62.

20. Frith D, Brohi K. The pathophysiology of trauma-induced coagulopathy. Curr Opin Crit Care 2012;18(6):631–6.

21. Holcomb JB, Wade CE, Michalek JE, et al. Increased plasma and platelet to red blood cell ratios improves outcome in 466 massively transfused civilian trauma patients. Ann Surg 2008;248:447–58.

22. Sperry JL, Ochoa JB, Gunn SR, et al. An FFP: RBC transfusion ratio >/=1:1.5 is associated with lower risk of mortality after massive transfusion. J Trauma 2008;65:986–93.

23. Perkins JG, Cap AP, Spinella PC, et al. An evaluation of the impact of apheresis platelets used in the setting of massively transfused trauma patients. J Trauma 2009;66(4 Suppl):S77–84.

24. Shaz BH, Dente CJ, Nicholas J, et al. Increased number of coagulation products in relationship to red blood cell products transfused improves mortality in trauma patients. Transfusion 2010;50:493–500.

25. Holcomb JB, Zarzabal LA, Michalek JE, et al. Increased platelet:RBC ratios are associated with improved survival after massive transfusion. J Trauma 2011;71(2 Suppl 3):S318–28.

26. Ho AM, Dion PW, Yeung JH, et al. Prevalence of survivor bias in observational studies on fresh frozen plasma:erythrocyte ratios in trauma requiring massive transfusions. Anesthesiology 2012;116(3):716–28.

27. Holcomb JB, del Junco DJ, Fox EE, et al, PROMMTT Study Group. The prospective, observational, multicenter, major trauma transfusion (PROMMTT) study: comparative effectiveness of a time varying treatment with competing risks. JAMA Surg 2013;148(2):127–36.

28. Kashuk JL, Moore EE, Wohlauer M, et al. Initial experiences with point-of-care rapid thrombelastography for management of life-threatening post injury coagulopathy. Transfusion 2012;52(1):23–33.

29. Da Luz LT, Nascimento B, Shankarakutty AK, et al. Effect of thromboelastography (TEG®) and rotational thromboelastometry (ROTEM®) on diagnosis of coagulopathy transfusion guidance and mortality in trauma: descriptive systematic review. Crit Care 2014;18(5):518.

30. Morse BC, Dente CJ, Hodgman EI, et al. The effects of protocolized use of recombinant factor VIIa within a massive transfusion protocol in a civilian level I trauma center. Am Surg 2011;77(8):1043–9.

31. Henry DA, Carless PA, Moxey AJ, et al. Anti-fibrinolytic use for minimizing perioperative allogeneic blood transfusion. Cochrane Database Syst Rev 2011;(3):CD001886.

32. Shakur H, Roberts I, Bautista R, et al. Effects of tranexamic acid on death, vascular occlusive events, and blood transfusion in trauma patients with significant haemorrhage (CRASH-2): a randomized, placebo-controlled trial. Lancet 2010;376:23–32.

33. Burgess AR, Eastridge BJ, Young JW, et al. Pelvic ring disruptions: effective classification system and treatment protocols. J Trauma 1990;30:848–56.

34. Starr AJ, Griffin DR, Reinert CM, et al. Pelvic ring disruptions: Prediction of associated injuries, transfusion requirement, pelvic arteriography, complications and mortality. J Orthop Trauma 2002;16:553–61.

35. Eastridge BJ, Starr A, Minei JP, et al. The importance of fracture pattern in guiding therapeutic decision-making in patients with hemorrhagic shock and pelvic ring disruptions. J Trauma 2002;53(3):446–50.

36. Hou Z, Smith WR, Strohecker KA, et al. Hemodynamically unstable pelvic fracture management by Advanced Trauma Life Support guidelines results in high mortality. Orthopedics 2012;35(3):e319–24.

37. Agolini SF, Shah K, Jaffe J, et al. Arterial embolization is a rapid and effective technique for controlling pelvic fracture hemorrhage. J Trauma 1997;43:395–9.

38. Balogh Z, Caldwell E, Heetveld M, et al. Institutional practice guidelines on management of pelvic fracture-related hemodynamic instability: do they make a difference? J Trauma 2005;58: 778–82.

39. Pohlmann T, Gansslen A, Bosch U, et al. The technique of packing for control of hemorrhage in complex pelvic fractures. Tech Orthop 1995;9: 267–70.

40. Ertel W, Keel M, Eid K, et al. Control of severe hemorrhage using C-clamp and pelvic packing in multiply injured patients with pelvic ring disruption. J Orthop Trauma 2001;15:468–74.

41. Cothren CC, Osborn PM, Moore EE, et al. Preperitoneal Pelvic packing for hemodynamically unstable pelvic fractures: a paradigm shift. J Trauma 2007;62:834–42.

42. Cothren Burlew CC, Moore EE, Smith WR, et al. Preperitoneal pelvic packing/external fixation with secondary angioembolization: optimal care for life-threatening hemorrhage from unstable pelvic fractures. J Am Coll Surg 2011;212(4): 628–35.

43. Smith W, Williams A, Agudelo J, et al. Early predictors of mortality in hemodynamically unstable pelvis fractures. J Orthop Trauma 2007; 21:31–7.

44. Vincent JL, Dufaye P, Berre J, et al. Serial lactate determinations during circulatory shock. Crit Care Med 1983;11:449–51.

45. Abramson D, Scalea TM, Hitchcock R, et al. Lactate clearance and survival following injury. J Trauma 1993;45:584–9.

46. Manikis P, Jankowski S, Zhang H, et al. Correlation of serial blood lactate levels to organ failure and mortality after trauma. Am J Emerg Med 1995;13: 619–22.

47. Siegel JH. Immediate versus delayed fluid resuscitation in patients with trauma. N Engl J Med 1995;332:681.

48. Davis JW, Parks SN, Kaups KL, et al. Admission base deficit predicts transfusion requirements and risk of complications. J Trauma 1996;41:769–74.

49. Davis JW, Kaups KL, Parks SN. Base deficit is superior to pH in evaluating clearance of acidosis after traumatic shock. J Trauma 1998;44:114–8.

50. Mikulaschek A, Henry SM, Donovan R, et al. Serum lactate is not predicted by anion gap or base excess after trauma resuscitation. J Trauma 1996; 40:218–22.

51. Paladino L, Sinert R, Wallace D, et al. The utility of base deficit and arterial lactate in differentiating major from minor injury in trauma patients with normal vital signs. Resuscitation 2008;77:363–8.

Pediatrics

Pediatric Open Fractures

Arianna Trionfo, MD[a],*, Priscilla K. Cavanaugh, MD[b],
Martin J. Herman, MD[b]

KEYWORDS

- Pediatric fractures • Open fracture • Pediatric trauma • Irrigation and debridement
- Type 1 open fracture

KEY POINTS

- Open fractures pose a risk for contamination and can lead to significant complications in children.
- These fractures often have a better prognosis in children as compared with adults.
- Open fractures in children differ from open fractures in adults, with faster and more reliable bone healing, greater potential for periosteal bone formation, and lower reported infection rates.

INTRODUCTION

Open fractures are characterized by disruption of the skin and underlying soft tissues due to either a penetrating wound or a displaced bone fragment resulting in direct communication between the fracture and the external environment.[1] These injuries are considered orthopedic emergencies because they are at high risk for contamination, potentially causing infection and significant morbidity. Open fractures constitute between 0.7% and 2% of all pediatric fractures.[2–4] In a recent retrospective study of pediatric fractures admitted to 2 tertiary care centers, 33 of 2840 (1%) of all fractures were open.[4] Most pediatric open fractures are a result of high-energy mechanisms, such as falls from heights and motor vehicle accidents. Although demographics and injury mechanisms vary widely, most studies report a higher incidence in male patients.[3,4] A multicenter study of 554 pediatric open fractures by Skaggs and colleagues[5] found the most common sites of injury were the fibula or tibia (190/554 fractures; 34%), ulna or radius (178/554; 32%), and hand or metacarpals (54/554; 10%).

Pediatric open fractures differ from adult open fractures in a variety of ways. Young children possess greater fracture stability and experience more rapid and reliable fracture healing compared with adults because of a thicker, more vascular periosteum.[6] In addition, children heal faster, have a greater potential for periosteal bone formation, and regenerate bone more easily in the setting of bone loss.[7,8] Children also have lower reported open fracture infection rates as compared with adults.[9] These differences are important to consider when managing open fractures in children. The purpose of this article is to review the initial evaluation and management and the definitive treatment options for pediatric open fractures.

INITIAL EVALUATION AND MANAGEMENT

Primary Survey and Resuscitation

The initial assessment of children with open fractures begins with performing a primary survey, which consists of the ABCs (airway, breathing, and circulation), a brief neurologic examination, and complete patient exposure.[10,11] In addition, the cervical spine should be stabilized to protect the child with a potential cervical spine injury, taking care to avoid neck flexion.[12]

Conflicts of Interest: The authors declare no conflicts of interest.
[a] Department of Orthopaedic Surgery, Temple University School of Medicine, 3401 North Broad Street, Philadelphia, PA 19140, USA; [b] Department of Orthopaedic Surgery, St. Christopher's Hospital for Children, Drexel University College of Medicine, 160 East Erie Avenue, Philadelphia, PA 19134, USA
* Corresponding author.
E-mail address: atrionfo1@gmail.com

Initial resuscitation of pediatric trauma patients follows the PALS (pediatric advanced life support) and ATLS (advanced trauma life support) guidelines.[13,14] On arrival into the trauma bay, intravenous access should be obtained, and intravenous fluids should be promptly administered.[15] For the patient with an obvious open fracture, intravenous antibiotics are also given (see Table 3).

Secondary Survey

Once the primary survey is completed and the resuscitation process has been initiated, a secondary survey that includes a thorough history and physical examination is conducted. The history should include confirmation of the patient's tetanus status. For all patients with an obvious open fracture, a dose of tetanus toxoid (0.5 mL intramuscular injection) is administered to patients who have not received a tetanus immunization within the past 5 years or if their status is unknown[12] (Table 1). Inspection, palpation, neurologic and vascular examination should be performed on all extremities. Compartments should be palpated to ensure that they are soft and compressible. Compartment syndrome should be suspected if compartments are tense, if the patient is reporting severe and escalating pain, and if passive stretch of the digits causes a significant increase in pain, among other signs. If suspected, compartment pressures should be measured promptly.

The open wound is inspected for bleeding, obvious injury to underlying structures, crush injuries to the soft tissues, bone exposure, and contamination. A sterile dressing is applied after wound assessment and bedside irrigation. Repeat wound inspections requiring dressing changes are minimized to avoid additional contamination risk and soft tissue injury. Before the patient is taken for advanced imaging or to the operating room, extremities with gross deformity should be realigned with gentle traction and splinted to minimize soft tissue injury and decrease pain.

Damage Control Orthopedics

Open fractures in children are often associated with polytrauma. In a retrospective study of children with open fractures, Cullen and colleagues[16] found that 58% (48/83) of the children in this series had other major injuries. Robertson and colleagues[17] reported that 82% (9/11) of children with an open femur fracture and 56% (18/32) with an open tibia fracture had associated injuries. In addition, the open fracture itself may be significantly unstable or involve extensive soft tissue injury. For these complicated cases, damage control orthopedics has been suggested. Damage control orthopedics is a well-recognized concept in adult orthopedic trauma that advocates for temporary fracture stabilization with external fixation until the patient is medically stabilized enough to allow for definitive fracture treatment.[18] Damage control orthopedics is based on the philosophy that early definitive fixation acts as a second major physiologic stressor ("second hit") that may be detrimental to a critically injured patient already affected by a significant injury ("first hit").[18]

There is a paucity of literature demonstrating the use of damage control orthopedics in pediatrics. However, the delay of definitive surgery in critically ill pediatric patients is practical in certain situations. At the authors' institution, a damage control protocol is used for children with

1. A traumatic brain injury with intracranial pressure measuring greater than 30 mm Hg despite medical intervention;
2. Persistent hemodynamic instability despite resuscitation efforts;
3. The "triad of death" (acidosis, hypothermia, and coagulopathy).

Table 1				
Tetanus prophylaxis recommendations				
	Clean, Minor Wounds		**All Other Wounds[a]**	
Vaccination History	**Td[b]**	**TIG**	**Td[b]**	**TIG**
Unknown or <3	Yes	No	Yes	Yes
≥3	Only if last dose >10 y	No	Only if last dose >5 y	No

Abbreviations: Td, tetanus and diphtheria; TIG, tetanus immune globulin.
   [a] Wounds >1 cm, incurred >6 h earlier, crush injuries, devitalized tissue, gross contamination with dirt, feces, and other.
   [b] If patient is <7 years old, give DTaP (diphtheria, tetanus, and pertussis). If patient is between 7 and 10 years old, give Td. Older children, give Tdap (tetanus, diphtheria, and pertussis).

CLASSIFICATION

The modified Gustilo and Anderson classification system is used for the classification of open fractures in both adults and children (Table 2).[19,20] A type I open fracture is a low-energy puncture wound less than 1 cm in length, with minimal soft tissue injury, fracture comminution, or contamination. Type II open fractures have wounds measuring 1 to 10 cm, without significant periosteal stripping or comminution, and have soft tissue quality adequate for wound coverage. Type III open fractures include subtypes A, B, and C. A type IIIA open fracture has adequate soft tissue coverage despite having a heavily contaminated wound measuring greater than 10 cm, and segmental or comminuted fractures. Type IIIB fractures have extensive soft tissue damage requiring coverage procedures typically associated with periosteal stripping, exposed bone, and significant contamination. Type IIIC open fractures have an associated vascular injury requiring immediate repair. In general, low-energy gunshot wounds are not classified as open fractures and may be safely treated nonoperatively. However, high-energy wounds mandate immediate and aggressive treatment that follows an open fracture protocol.[21]

On initial examination, the extent of soft tissue injury tends to be underestimated. It has been shown that stage diagnosed at the time of debridement often differs from the initial preoperative classification, with definitive staging more accurately done in the operating room.[22] It is particularly important in small children to focus not on the length of the wound but, more importantly, on the extent of soft tissue damage and periosteal stripping. Regardless, initial staging should be performed expeditiously and as accurately as possible because it dictates the initial choice of antibiotic therapy.

OPEN FRACTURE MANAGEMENT

Successful outcomes can be expected in most pediatric patients with open fractures by adhering to basic principles of open fracture management and applying them in every case.

PREVENTION OF INFECTION

Factors Influencing Infection

Most pediatric open fractures are potentially contaminated at the time of injury, increasing the risk of subsequent wound infection. Infection rates based on the Gustilo-Anderson fracture type in children vary, but generally type III fractures have been associated with higher infection rates compared with type I and II fractures. In a study of 44 pediatric open femur fractures by Hutchins and colleagues,[23] infections were associated with type III open fractures (5/10), but not with the type I (0/25) or type II (0/9) fractures. A retrospective study of 554 pediatric open fractures reported a 3% overall infection rate, with an incidence of 2% (5/302) in type I fractures, 2% (3/154) in type II fractures, and 8% (8/98) in type III fractures.[5] In addition, age has been reported to be correlated with infection rate in open fractures. In a retrospective study of 31 pediatric open fractures, Blaiser and Barnes[24] demonstrated that children 12 years of age or older had a higher infection rate compared with those younger than 12 years old, with rates of 31% and 7% ($P = .065$), respectively. Therefore, it may be important to distinguish between younger and older children when determining open fracture infection risk.

Antibiotic Therapy

Prompt administration of prophylactic antibiotic therapy decreases the risk of infection in children with open fractures. In the study of 1104 open fractures by Patzakis and Wilkins,[9] an infection rate of 7.4% (49/661) was reported when

Table 2	
The Gustilo and Anderson classification of open fractures	
Type	**Definition**
I	Wound <1 cm; minimal contamination, soft tissue damage, no comminution
II	Wound >1 cm; moderate soft tissue damage, minimal periosteal stripping
IIIA	Wound >10 cm; extensive soft tissue damage, substantial contamination, adequate coverage
IIIB	Wound >10 cm; extensive soft tissue damage, substantial contamination, inadequate coverage
IIIC	Wound >10 cm; extensive soft tissue damage, vascular injury requiring repair

Adapted from Gustilo RB, Mendoza RM, Williams DN. Problems in the management of type III (severe) open fractures: a new classification of type III open fractures. J Trauma 1984;24:742–6; and Melvin JS, Dombroski DG, Torbert JT, et al. Open tibial shaft fractures: I. Evaluation and initial wound management. J Am Acad Orthop Surg 2010;18(1):10–9.

antibiotics were started more than 3 hours after injury and 4.7% (17/364) when antibiotics were started within 3 hours after injury. The investigators concluded that the single most important factor in reducing infection rate in these patients was early administration of antibiotics.[9] Today, most surgeons agree that prophylactic antibiotics should be started as soon as possible.

Although there is a strong consensus on the timely initial administration of antibiotics, the ideal duration of therapy remains somewhat controversial. A randomized, double-blind prospective trial by Dellinger and colleagues[25] compared a 1-day versus 5-day course of postoperative antibiotics in 248 patients with open fractures. No reduction in infection rates was found with the longer 5-day versus 1-day course of cefonicid (13% vs 12%, respectively).[25] These findings were consistent across all 3 Gustilo-Anderson types of open fractures. However, it is important to note that patients less than the age of 14 were excluded from this study. Currently, many investigators advise that initial antibiotic prophylaxis should be limited to a 24- to 72-hour course.[26,27] Skaggs and colleagues recommend administration of antibiotics for 24 hours after wound closure; at the authors' institution, children with open fractures typically receive 48 hours of antibiotic therapy.

Antibiotic Selection

A first-generation cephalosporin is typically administered to patients with an open fracture (see **Table 3**). In the classic study by Patzakis and colleagues,[28] 3 groups of patients with open fractures were randomized to receive placebo, penicillin and streptomycin, or cephalothin. Infection rates were 13.9%, 9.7%, and 2.3%, respectively.[28] This finding provided evidence for the use of cephalosporins directed against gram-positive organisms in open fractures and has since been supported in the literature.[25] Patients with type II or III open fractures are additionally given an aminoglycoside to enhance gram-negative coverage. Penicillin or one of its derivatives is added to cover anaerobes and *Clostridium* species when dealing with dirty wounds, such as those exposed to soil. Patients allergic to cephalosporins or penicillin are commonly given clindamycin. The increasing incidence of community-acquired methicillin-resistant *Staphylococcus aureus* (MRSA) has led to the concern that traditional prophylactic antibiotic recommendations may not be sufficient. However, the benefits of prophylactic regimens against MRSA have not been established in the literature, and currently, there is a paucity of high-quality studies that support the routine use of clindamycin, vancomycin, or other antibiotics instead of cephalosporins for pediatric open fracture prophylaxis. Therefore, the decision to include MRSA coverage for pediatric open fracture prophylaxis is made by the surgeon and should be based on individualized risk factors.

Local antibiotic therapy has been shown to be valuable in the prevention of infection in open fractures when used as an adjunct to systemic antibiotics.[29] Antibiotic-laden polymethylmethacrylate (PMMA) beads are commonly used and have been shown to decrease infection risk of severe type III open fractures in adults. In a retrospective study of 1085 open tibial fractures, Ostermann and colleagues[29] found an infection rate of 3.7% in patients treated with both gentamicin bead chains and systemic antibiotics compared with a 12% infection rate for those that received systemic antibiotics alone (P<.001). In a more recent study of 75 open fractures, patients were randomized to receive either traditional systemic antibiotics or antibiotic-PMMA bead chains. Infection occurred in 5.3% (2/38) of fractures treated only with systemic antibiotics and in 8.3% (2/24) of those

Table 3		
Antibiotic therapy for pediatric open fractures		
Antibiotic	**Pediatric Dose**	**Indication**
Cefazolin (Ancef)	25–100 mg/kg/dose every 8 h	All open fractures
Clindamycin	25–40 mg/kg/d every 6-8 h	PCN or cephalosporin allergy
Gentamicin	5–7.5 mg/kg/d every 8 h	Type II and III open fractures
Penicillin	50,000–100,000 units/kg IV every 4 h	Soil/fecal contamination
Vancomycin	15 mg/kg/dose every 6 h	Suspected MRSA infections

Abbreviations: IV, intravenous; PCN, penicillin.

From Rosenblatt J, et al. Open tibia fractures in children and adolescents. In: Abzug JM, Herman MJ, editors. Pediatric Orthopaedic surgical emergencies. 1st edition. New York: Springer Scoenve + Business Media; 2012. p. 161; with permission.

treated only with antibiotic bead chains.[30] These findings suggest that although antibiotic beads may provide protection against infection, they should not be considered a substitute for systemic therapy. Moreover, antibiotic-PMMA bead chains may be most useful in the setting of open fractures with extensive bone loss, where they provide local therapy and occupy dead space that would otherwise serve as a potential nidus for infection before definitive surgery can be performed.[31] Unfortunately, there is a paucity of literature on the use of antibiotic beads for the treatment of pediatric open fractures, and the decision to use them should be made on a case-by-case basis. It is important to note, however, that local antibiotic therapy is generally considered safe and that high local antibiotic concentrations with low systemic levels are often achieved.[32]

Topical vancomycin powder has shown efficacy in decreasing postoperative infections in spine surgery, but has not yet been fully studied in open fracture surgery. Singh and colleagues[33] conducted a retrospective review assessing the efficacy of vancomycin powder in reducing surgical site infection (SSI) rates in adult patients with high-energy tibial plateau and pilon fractures, which included 83 patients in the control group (23/83; 28% with open fractures) and 10 (3/10; 30% open fractures) in the vancomycin group. There was no statistically significant difference in the rate of SSI between the vancomycin group, 10% (1/10), and the control group, 16.7% (14/83).[33] Moreover, it is unknown whether the infected cases were open or closed fractures. There is a clear need for studies to delineate the role of vancomycin powder as a modality to reduce postoperative infection in pediatric open fractures.

TIMING OF SURGERY

In the treatment of open fractures, traditional teaching is that all open fractures must be treated by irrigation and debridement within 6 to 8 hours from the time of injury. Although this practice is widely accepted, little evidence supports it. In fact, several current studies in children have demonstrated no significant difference in infection rates when surgery was delayed for greater than 6 hours and even as long as 24 hours after injury as long as intravenous antibiotics are started on presentation.[5,34] Therefore, irrigation and debridement of pediatric open fractures can be performed within the first 24 hours after injury without significantly increasing the risk for infection, provided antibiotics are given early. However, emergent surgery should be considered in cases involving gross contamination, vascular compromise of the extremity, large bone exposure, and severe soft tissue injury.

IRRIGATION AND DEBRIDEMENT

Thorough irrigation and debridement is the sine qua non of open fracture treatment. The open wound is extended to permit adequate exposure of the fracture fragments and surrounding soft tissue. Although the need for debridement of devitalized tissue and gross contaminants has never been called into question, initial debridement in children should be more conservative than that of similar wounds in an adult population. In the pediatric population, it is recommended that fracture fragments with questionable viability and a soft tissue attachment be retained because they may incorporate into the fracture union.

The Orthopaedic Trauma Association has established guidelines for the amount of irrigation recommended for adult open fractures; however, there is no standard recommendation for children. Instead, the volume of irrigation in a pediatric population must be tailored to match both the size of the wound and the patient's limb as well as the degree of contamination. Irrigation volume in a pediatric population rarely exceeds 5 L. Excessive irrigation, especially when delivered under high pressure, may extravasate into soft tissues and theoretically increase the risk for compartment syndrome as well as impede bone healing.[35] Studies have shown that the addition of antibiotics to irrigation does not lessen the risk of infection and may have a deleterious effect on wound healing.[36–38] In contrast, the addition of a gentle soap or detergent may be more effective in removing bacteria from bone.[37]

WOUND MANAGEMENT

Common practice involves avoiding primary closure of open wounds after initial debridement in order to allow an outlet for any possible retained nidus of infection. However, in recent years, wound management strategies have become less dogmatic. Recent evidence suggests that it is safe to close a low-grade traumatic wound over a drain if there is no gross contamination and the soft tissues appear healthy and viable.[16] At the authors' institution, most grade I and II wounds that appear clean after irrigation and can be reapproximated without tension are closed primarily, often over a drain. If a second debridement is indicated, the wound is reopened, debrided, and closed. Type III injuries, by definition, defy primary closure, and local or remote flap coverage may be necessary after all underlying tissue is deemed viable. A popular alternative treatment for wound coverage is the use of a vacuum-assisted wound closure (VAC) device. This technique has been found to provide notable advantages over traditional wound care in younger patients and may even preclude the need for tissue transfer in some cases. Patients require fewer painful dressing changes, and the risk of wound contamination is diminished because the wound is sealed. It is hypothesized that the VAC system may reduce soft tissue edema and promote granulation tissue by removing debris and soluble inflammatory mediators that inhibit wound healing.[39] In a retrospective review of 28 pediatric patients with 37 diverse open fractures initially treated with wound VAC therapy, 5.4% (2/37) were found to have a deep infection.[40] The investigators concluded that when compared with historical controls, the use of VAC therapy seemed equally effective and safe in reducing infection risk in pediatric open fractures. The authors generally apply the VAC to larger wounds that have questionably viable tissue after debridement or were grossly contaminated at initial surgery. The VAC is changed every other day until the wound can be closed primarily or, in cases with large soft tissue defects, is ready for plastic surgery coverage.

FRACTURE STABILIZATION

Stabilization of an open fracture is essential to reduce pain, prevent additional injury to surrounding soft tissues, decrease inflammatory response, and promote early mobilization. In the pediatric population, methods of stabilization are varied depending on patient age, location and severity of the fracture, and extent of soft tissue injury. The choice of fixation must also take into account access to the limb for wound and neurovascular evaluations as well as future needs for soft tissue management. Closed reduction and cast immobilization may be used for grade I open injuries that have stable fracture configurations after reduction.

Humeral Fractures
Open fractures of the humeral shaft and the supracondylar humerus are uncommon in childhood with a reported rate of 0.5% to 1% of all

forearm fractures.[41] In one series of 15 patients with open supracondylar or humeral shaft fractures, the investigators reported 13% arterial injury, 47% nerve injury, but overall 85% excellent or good outcomes when treated with antibiotics, irrigation, and debridement within 12 hours of injury and fracture fixation.[41] Stabilization methods for open diaphyseal humeral fractures include intramedullary flexible nailing or compression plating. External fixation is an option in patients with severe soft tissue injury and gross contamination. Typically, lateral-entry Kirschner-wire fixation provides adequate fixation for open supracondylar fractures. Overall, infection rate in this population remains low, likely because of the highly collateralized blood flow around the elbow in children.

Forearm Fractures
Open forearm and wrist fractures account for approximately 1% to 2%% of all pediatric forearm fractures.[42,43] In recent years, there has been a trend to treat open forearm fractures with surgical fixation, as opposed to closed reduction and cast immobilization. This trend towards operative management is based on evidence to suggest that fracture stabilization minimizes the risk of nonunion and malunion, while at the same time maintaining a low rate of infectious complications.[41,44,45] Percutaneous Kirschner-wire fixation (Fig. 1) typically provides adequate stability for fractures of the distal radius and ulna, while flexible intramedullary nails are commonly used for diaphyseal forearm fractures. Although internal fixation is the current trend, Lim and colleagues[46] reported a series of patients with grade I and II open forearm fractures treated with cast immobilization and compared them with patients treated with internal fixation. Both groups had 100% excellent or good results, and there was no significant difference in time to union. This study serves as a reminder that internal fixation for open forearm fractures is not a foregone conclusion and that some of these injuries may be successfully treated with casting after irrigation and debridement.

Femoral Fractures
Open femur fractures are rare but severe injuries that are caused by high-energy mechanisms to breach the large soft tissue compartment surrounding the femur. They account for approximately 4% of all pediatric femur fractures.[23] Although the optimal method of fracture stabilization remains controversial, excellent functional results have been reported with various treatment methods. In one study from a large urban

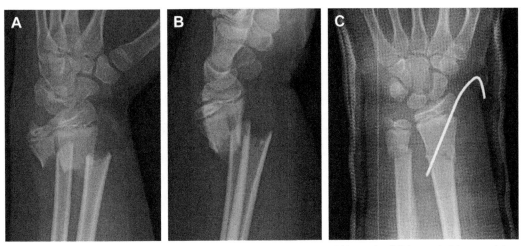

Fig. 1. (A) Anteroposterior (AP) and (B) lateral radiograph of a 14-year-old boy who fell from a ladder sustaining a grade I open distal radius and ulna fracture. (C) AP radiograph after irrigation, debridement, and percutaneous K-wire fixation. He went on to heal uneventfully.

pediatric trauma center, 44 open femoral fractures in 43 children were treated with a variety of modalities including spica casting, external fixation, locked intramedullary nailing, open reduction and plate fixation, and pins and plaster. The investigators concluded that type I and II fractures can typically be treated with irrigation and debridement followed by age-appropriate fixation methods. However, the optimal fixation for type III fractures remains unresolved.[23]

Many children less than 6 years of age may be treated with spica casting alone after thorough irrigation and debridement, assuming that the shortening of the fracture measured on the injury film or in the operating room is less than 2.5 to 3 cm.[23,47] However, this strategy may pose a problem for soft tissue management if repeated dressing changes or repeat surgical debridements are needed. Traditional plate fixation, or the less invasive technique of submuscular bridge plating, may be used to treat open diaphyseal femur fractures.[48,49] External fixation of open femoral shaft fractures was routinely used in the past because it allows easy access for wound care and is efficient when damage control techniques are used. However, because of a high delayed union and refracture rate, as well as an increased infection rate, the present trend is to use external fixation only for fractures that are not amenable to internal fixation because of their location, fracture pattern, or soft tissue considerations.[50,51]

Intramedullary nailing has become the preferred treatment for diaphyseal femur fractures in children, especially for those between 6 and 12 years of age (Fig. 2). Although most major series in children include both open and closed

femur fractures, intramedullary nailing with flexible or rigid locked nails may be used effectively to manage open femur fractures. Contraindications to the use of these devices include fracture patterns not amenable to intramedullary fixation, such as length unstable fracture patterns when using flexible nails, grossly contaminated wounds, and very proximal or very distal femoral fractures. In several series of children with open femoral shaft fractures, patients who were treated with intramedullary fixation versus external fixator had quicker return to school, normal joint range of motion, and earlier mobilization than those treated with external fixation.[52,53]

Tibial Fractures

Open fractures of the tibia are rare, comprising only 2% to 3% of all tibia fractures. However, open tibia fractures account for approximately one-third of all open fractures in children.[5] Successful treatment of open tibial fractures in patients with open physes has been achieved with percutaneous pinning in young children, external fixation, flexible intramedullary nail fixation, and plate constructs. Older adolescents with a nearly fused tibial tubercle may be treated as adults with reamed, locked, intramedullary nailing.

External fixation is the traditional fixation method for management of open fractures with severe comminution, with segmental bone loss, and in medically unstable patients. It has been shown to yield satisfactory results in patients with type II and III tibial shaft fractures, including those with butterfly fragments.[54] Although the devices are easy to apply and are familiar to most orthopedic surgeons, external

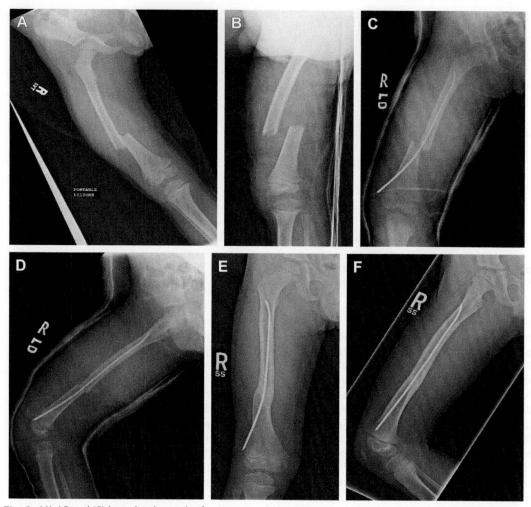

Fig. 2. (A) AP and (B) lateral radiograph of an 11-year-old boy after an all-terrain vehicle accident. He sustained grade 3A open femur fracture. (C, D) In attempting to place the medial rod, the cortex was broken, so he was placed in a spica cast with a single rod to maintain length. (E, F) AP and lateral radiographs at 9 months showing healed and remodeled fracture. His rod was removed.

fixation is not without complications, including deep infections, pin-track infections, delayed union, and refracture.[55,56]

Flexible intramedullary nails (Fig. 3) are the treatment of choice for many open tibial diaphyseal fractures in children because they do not cross the physes, maintain length and alignment, do not obstruct wound care, and permit rapid mobilization.[57] Several reports show flexible intramedullary nails to have good results. One retrospective review of both open and closed pediatric tibial fractures found that time to union was significantly shorter with elastic nails than with external fixation (7 vs 18 weeks, respectively). Functional outcome, including pain, happiness, return to sports, and global function, was also significantly better in the flexible nail

group.[58] However, flexible nails are less likely to yield satisfactory results for fractures within 2 to 3 cm of the physes, within length-unstable fractures, or for fractures occurring in patients weighing more than 100 lbs (45 kg).[59]

Percutaneous pinning of tibial shaft fractures is an option for very distal or proximal fractures, or for shaft fractures in very young children. However, one report that included 40 open tibial fractures that were treated percutaneously with Steinmann pins and supplemental casting showed a 23% delayed union and 10% malunion.[16] Plate and screw fixation is not commonly used for open tibia fractures because of the increased risk of infection. However, a recent retrospective review of 14 patients treated with minimally invasive percutaneous osteosynthesis

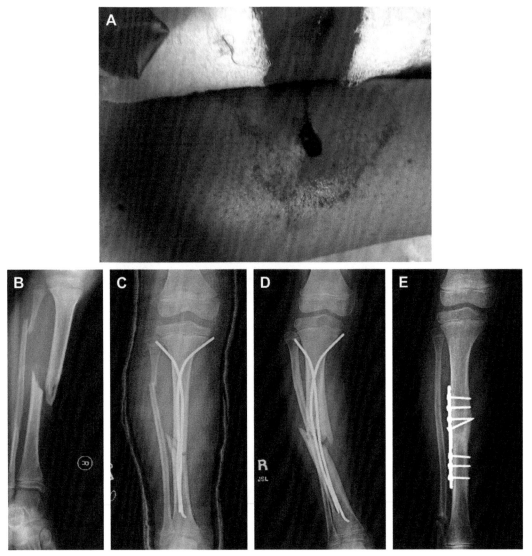

Fig. 3. (A) Clinical photograph and (B) AP radiograph of a 12-year-old boy struck by a motor vehicle. He sustained a grade 3A tibial shaft fracture. (C) He underwent irrigation, debridement, and placement of flexible nails. (D) He had been lost to follow-up and returned 6 months after the injury complaining of deformity and was found to have an aseptic nonunion. (E) AP radiograph taken 4 months after he underwent excision of callous and iliac crest bone grafting of the incomplete union with plate fixation.

(MIPO) showed good results. All fractures healed with a mean time to union of 18 weeks. There were no reported infections, malunion, or limb length discrepancy observed. The investigators advocate that MIPO may be an effective alternative treatment of open pediatric tibial fractures.[60]

Open tibia fractures are the most challenging of all pediatric open fractures. By adhering to the basic principles of open fracture management, restoration of normal function can be expected in nearly all cases (Fig. 4). In general, however, patients less than the age of 12 years heal faster and have lower infection rates and fewer complications than older children with open tibia fractures.[55,61] Children greater than the age of 12 years tend to have complication rates similar to those of adults.[62]

Pelvic Fracture
Pelvic fractures are uncommon in children, with open pelvic injuries being exceedingly rare. In one retrospective review of 15 pediatric patients with open pelvic fractures treated at a single institution, investigators showed that most

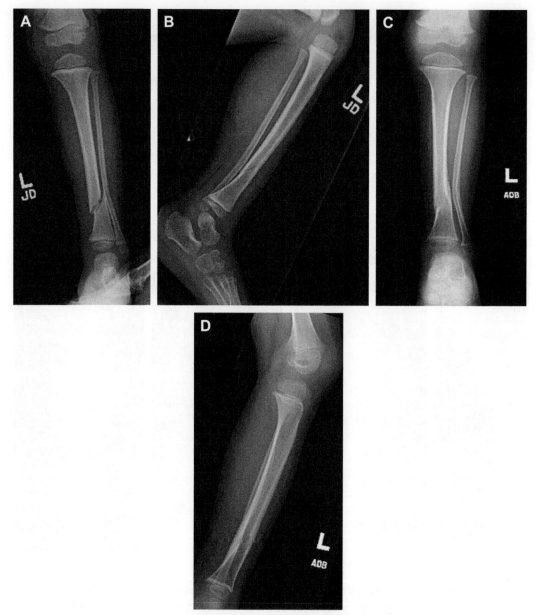

Fig. 4. (A) AP and (B) lateral radiograph of a 6-year-old boy with a grade 2 open tibia fracture. (C) AP and (D) lateral radiograph 8 weeks after treatment with irrigation, debridement, closed reduction, and casting.

(10/15) had vertically unstable fracture patterns resulting from high-energy mechanisms. Three of 15 patients died, with sepsis and infection from concomitant bowel and bladder injuries being the most common complications.[63] Although the open wound is obvious in some cases, fracture fragments may lacerate the vaginal wall in female patients, disrupt the urethra, and injure the bowel, causing contamination that may not be readily apparent. Patients with unstable open pelvic fractures are best treated with antibiotics, debridement of open wounds, and fracture fixation to maintain a stable pelvic ring and limit internal bleeding, ongoing soft tissue, and viscus injury. External fixation provides provisional stability while allowing abdominal access in patients with multiple injuries and can serve either as definitive fixation or as a bridge to more definitive internal fixation techniques. In addition, diverting colostomies and cystostomies should be used as needed to manage injuries and diminish the risk of infection.

Foot Fractures

Lawnmower-associated trauma is responsible for a significant number of life-altering injuries in children and adolescents. Several series of children seen with lawnmower injuries note a 30% to 50% amputation rate.[64,65] Most nonamputation injuries involve the lower extremity and foot.[65] These injuries typically require a multidisciplinary approach with multiple trips to the operating room for irrigation, debridement, and extensive soft tissue coverage.

Fractures of the distal phalangeal growth plate with overlying nail bed laceration are termed Seymour fractures.[66] Because of the overlying nail bed disruption, these injuries are technically considered open fractures. Seymour fractures may occur in the fingers or the toes and may lead to significant morbidity if not recognized and appropriately debrided. In one retrospective review of 5 patients with open fractures of the great toe distal phalanx, no infection occurred in those that were recognized early and treated with antibiotics. However, 3 children with delayed diagnoses and treatment developed osteomyelitis.[67] A recent retrospective case series of 24 patients with Seymour fractures in the upper extremity included 9 patients with closed injuries that were treated nonoperatively and 15 patients with open injuries that underwent surgical management. Of the patients treated nonoperatively, 3 received oral antibiotics because they had severe soft tissue damage and because treatment began more than 6 hours after injury. All patients who underwent surgical management received preoperative and postoperative antibiotics No infections occurred in either group.[68] These results lend credence to the importance of early recognition and treatment.

Management of Seymour fractures involves removal of the nail plate and any interposed soft tissue in order to allow for accurate reduction. The fracture site must be thoroughly irrigated and the sterile matrix repaired with 5-0 or 6-0 chromic gut sutures. Often the nail plate or suture packaging material is placed under the eponychial fold. At this point, the fracture is often stable and does not require fixation. However, if the fracture remains unstable, retrograde K-wire fixation may be required.

CONTROVERSIES
Type I Open Fracture Management

Since before the publication of Gustillo and Anderson's landmark work, all open fractures were routinely treated with urgent irrigation and debridement. However, recent literature has challenged this dogma by calling into question the role of operative intervention for type I injuries. Two relatively recent retrospective studies demonstrated similar infection and outcome rates for patients treated with and without surgery for type I open fractures in children. One treatment protocol involved irrigation and debridement in the emergency department followed by 24 hours of intravenous antibiotic administration in the inpatient hospital setting and reported a 2.5% infection rate. They treated a total of 40 open fractures, including 8 tibia fractures, 18 diaphyseal forearm fractures, and 14 distal radius and ulna fractures.[69] The other protocol involved treating patients in a similar manner but either discharging patients home with an oral antibiotic or admitting them for less than 24 hours, reporting a 4% infection rate. They treated a total of 25 open fractures including 18 both-bone forearm fractures, 2 Monteggia fractures, and 5 tibial shaft fractures.[70] In the most recent retrospective review of 40 pediatric forearm and tibia type I open fractures treated nonoperatively, Bazzi and colleagues[71] showed that there were no infections and only one delayed union. These studies suggest that nonoperative treatment of type I open fractures in a pediatric population may be safe and have little risk of infection.[71]

Critics of the nonoperative approach to type I open fractures have voiced several concerns about the safety of such an approach. These published studies are all grossly underpowered, making conclusions drawn from this data difficult to interpret. More importantly, it is the experience of some that foreign bodies and organic material may be introduced into a grade I wound, regardless of how minor it appears. Finally, gas gangrene from clostridium contamination can cause limb- and life-threatening sepsis. Many argue that surgical debridement for all open wounds regardless of grade is prudent in order to diminish the risk of this devastating infection.

At the authors' institution, the vast majority of grade I open fractures are treated with surgical debridement. The exceptions to this are some "inside-out" grade I injuries that occur after low- and middle-energy trauma without signs of gross contamination. All open fractures treated nonsurgically at the authors' institution receive antibiotics on admission, have the tetanus status addressed, undergo simple wound irrigation and sterile dressing application in the emergency department, and are admitted to the hospital for 48 hours of intravenous antibiotics. Anecdotally, they have used this protocol selectively for more than 15 years without major complications.

COMPLICATIONS

Delayed Bone Healing

Delayed healing and nonunions in pediatric open fractures are rare.[72] Tibial fractures are the most common source of pediatric nonunions, occurring in nearly 25% of immature patients with open tibial shaft fractures.[73] They tend to occur in older children and adolescents with less growth potential, in infected fractures, or in injuries with segmental bone loss or significant soft tissue stripping.[74,75] Open ulnar shaft fractures and ulnar fractures that require open reduction may show delayed healing after intramedullary fixation.[76] However, even in segmental fractures with bone loss, young children may have the osteogenic potential to replace a significant bone gap.[77]

The ideal treatment of delayed unions and nonunions is at times controversial and must be individualized. One must critically evaluate radiographs for signs of instability at the fracture site, such as progressive angulation, minimal callus formation, and radiographic lucency about fixator pin sites. Laboratory tests, including complete blood count, erythrocyte sedimentation rate, and C-reactive protein, should be obtained to rule out infection. The therapeutic principles of nonunion management in children involve excision of any interposed fibrous tissue, bone grafting, and stable fixation. Open reduction and internal fixation enhance union but do not guarantee it for all children.[75] As in the adult population, protected weight-bearing on the involved limb may enhance healing of delayed union in children. Despite anecdotal reports, no published data indicate that bone stimulators have been successful in treating tibial nonunion in children and adolescents. The Ilizarov fixator also has been reported to be useful in the management of these complications, especially for fractures with segmental defects.[74] It uses the principles of distraction histogenesis techniques to manage complicated defects and restore leg length. In addition, appropriate antibiotic treatment is necessary for patients with concomitant fracture sepsis.

SUMMARY

Open fractures in children are rare and present unique therapeutic challenges. Rapid administration of antibiotics is the sine qua non of infection prevention. Formal debridement is a long established principle in the treatment of open fractures, although timing to operative intervention and the need for debridement of type I open fractures remain controversial. Open fractures in children are typically associated with better prognoses compared with their adult equivalents. Fracture fixation is often used to help minimize soft tissue complications, but care must always be taken to preserve the physis of growing children.

REFERENCES

1. Dunbar RP, Gardner MJ. Chapter 10: Initial management of open fractures. In: Rockwood CA, Bucholz RV, Court-Brown CM, et al, editors. Fractures in adults. Philadelphia: Lippincott & Wilkins; 2010. p. 283–4.
2. Cheng JC, Ng BK, Ying SY, et al. A 10-year study of the changes in the pattern and treatment of 6,493 fractures. J Pediatr Orthop 1999;19(3):344–50.
3. Rennie L, Court-Brown CM, Mok JY, et al. The epidemiology of fractures in children. Injury 2007;38:913–22.
4. Joeris A, Lutz N, Wicki B, et al. An epidemiological evaluation of pediatric long bone fractures—a retrospective cohort study of 2716 patients from two Swiss tertiary pediatric hospitals. BMC Pediatr 2014;14:314.
5. Skaggs DL, Friend L, Alman B, et al. The effect of surgical delay on acute infection following 554 open fractures in children. J Bone Joint Surg Am 2005;87(1):8–12.
6. Rodriguez-Merchan EC. Pediatric skeletal trauma: a review and historical perspective. Clin Orthop Relat Res 2005;432:8–13.
7. Parfitt AM, Travers R, Rauch F, et al. Structural and cellular changes during bone growth in healthy children. Bone 2000;27:487–94.
8. Stewart DG, Kay RM, Skaggs DL. Open fractures in children. Principles of evaluation and management. J Bone Joint Surg Am 2005;87(12):2784–98.
9. Patzakis MJ, Wilkins J. Factors influencing infection rate in open fracture wounds. Clin Orthop Relat Res 1989;243:36–40.
10. Armstrong PF. Initial management of the multiply injured child: the ABC's. Instr Course Lect 1992;41:347–50.
11. Shires GT, Jones RC. Initial management of the severely injured patient. JAMA 1970;213:1872–8.
12. Abzug JM, Herman MJ. Polytrauma in the pediatric patient. In: Abzug JM, Herman MJ, editors. Pediatric orthopedic surgical emergencies. New York: Springer; 2012. p. 7–9.
13. American College of Surgeons, Committee on Trauma. Advanced trauma life support manual. Chicago: American College of Surgeons; 1997.

14. Chameides L, Hazinski MF, editors. Pediatric advanced life support. Dallas (TX): American Heart Association; 1997.

15. Guy J, Haley K, Zuspan SJ. Use of intraosseous infusion in the pediatric trauma patient. J Pediatr Surg 1993;28:158–61.

16. Cullen MC, Roy DR, Crawford AH, et al. Open fracture of the tibia in children. J Bone Joint Surg Am 1996;78:1039–47.

17. Robertson P, Karol LA, Rab GT. Open fractures of the tibia and femur in children. J Pediatr Orthop 1996;16:621–6.

18. Pape HC, Giannoudis P, Kretek C. The timing of fracture treatment in polytrauma patients: relevance of damage control orthopedic surgery. Am J Surg 2002;183:622–9.

19. Gustilo RB, Anderson JT. Prevention of infection in the treatment of one thousand and twenty-five open fractures of long bones: retrospective and prospective analyses. J Bone Joint Surg Am 1976; 58:453–8.

20. Gustilo RB, Mendoza RM, Williams DN. Problems in the management of type III (severe) open fractures: a new classification of type III open fractures. J Trauma 1984;24:742–6.

21. Bartlett CS, Helfet DL, Hausman MR, et al. Ballistics and gunshot wounds: effects on musculoskeletal tissues. J Am Acad Orthop Surg 2000;8(1):21–36.

22. Faraj AA. The reliability of the pre-operative classification of open tibial fractures in children a proposal for a new classification. Acta Orthop Belg 2002;68:49–55.

23. Hutchins CM, Sponseller PD, Sturm P, et al. Open femur fractures in children: treatment, complications, and results. J Pediatr Orthop 2000;20:183–8.

24. Blaiser RD, Barnes CL. Age as a prognostic factor in open tibial fractures in children. Clin Orthop Relat Res 1996;(331):262–4.

25. Dellinger EP, Caplan ES, Weaver LD, et al. Duration of preventive antibiotic administration for open extremity fractures. Arch Surg 1988;123(3):333–9.

26. Saveli CC, Belknap RW, Morgan SJ, et al. The role of prophylactic antibiotics in open fractures in an era of community-acquired methicillin-resistant Staphylococcus aureus. Orthopedics 2011;34(8): 611–6.

27. Melvin JS, Dombroski DG, Torbert JT, et al. Open tibial shaft fractures: I. Evaluation and initial wound management. J Am Acad Orthop Surg 2010;18(1): 10–9.

28. Patzakis MJ, Harvey JP Jr, Ivler D. The role of antibiotics in the management of open fractures. J Bone Joint Surg Am 1974;56:532–41.

29. Ostermann PA, Seligson D, Henry SL. Local antibiotic therapy for severe open fractures. A review of 1085 consecutive cases. J Bone Joint Surg Br 1995;77(1):93–7.

30. Moehring HD, Gravel C, Chapman MW, et al. Comparison of antibiotic beads and intravenous antibiotics in open fractures. Clin Orthop Relat Res 2000;372:254–61.

31. Ristiniemi J, Lakovaara M, Flinkkila T, et al. Staged method using antibiotic beads and subsequent autografting for large traumatic tibial bone loss: 22 of 23 fractures healed after 5-20 months. Acta Orthop 2007;78(4):520–7.

32. Zalavras CG, Patzakis MJ, Holtom P. Local antibiotic therapy in the treatment of open fractures and osteomyelitis. Clin Orthop Relat Res 2004;427:86–93.

33. Singh K, Baeuer JM, CaChaud GY, et al. Surgical site infection in high-energy peri-articular tibia fractures with intra-wound vancomycin powder: a retrospective pilot study. J Orthop Traumatol 2015; 16(4):287–91.

34. Skaggs L, Kautz SM, Kay RM, et al. Effect of delay of surgical treatment on rate of infection in open fractures in children. J Pediatr Orthop 2000;20:19–22.

35. Adili A, Bhandari M, Schemitsch EH. The biomechanical effects of highpressure irrigation on diaphyseal fracture healing in vivo. J Orthop Trauma 2002;16:413–7.

36. Anglen JO. Wound irrigation in musculoskeletal injury. J Am Acad Orthop Surg 2001;9:219–26.

37. Anglen JO. Comparison of soap and antibiotic solutions for irrigation of lower-limb open fracture wounds. J Bone Joint Surg Am 2005;87-A:1415–22.

38. Conroy BP, Anglen JO, Simpson W, et al. Comparison of castile soap, benzalkonium chloride, and bacitracin as irrigation solutions for complex contaminated orthopaedic wounds. J Orthop Trauma 1999;13:332–7.

39. Mooney JF, Argenta LC, Marks MW, et al. Treatment of soft tissue defects in pediatric patients using the V.A.C. system. Clin Orthop Relat Res 2000;376:26–31.

40. Halvorson J, Jinnah R, Kulp B, et al. Use of vacuum-assisted closure in pediatric open fractures with a focus on the rate of infection. Orthopedics 2011; 34:e256–60.

41. Haasbeek JF, Cole WG. Open fractures of the arm in children. J Bone Joint Surg Br 1995;77:576–81.

42. Flynn JM, Jones KJ, Garner MR, et al. Eleven years experience in the operative management of pediatric forearm fractures. J Pediatr Orthop 2010; 30(4):313–9.

43. Mehlman CT, Wall EJ. Rockwood and Wilkins' fractures in children. 7th edition. Philadelphia: Lippincott Williams and Wilkins; 2010. p. 328.

44. Luhmann SJ, Schootman M, Schoenecker PL, et al. Complications and outcomes of open pediatric forearm fractures. J Pediatr Orthop 2004;24:1–6.

45. Greenbaum B, Zionts LE, Ebramzadeh E. Open fractures of the forearm in children. J Orthop Trauma 2001;15:111–8.

46. Lim YJ, Lam KS, Lee EH. Open Gustilo 1 and 2 mid-shaft fractures of the radius and ulna in children: is there a role for cast immobilization after wound debridement? J Pediatr Orthop 2007;27:540–6.

47. Thompson JD, Buehler KC, Sponseller PD, et al. Shortening in femoral shaft fractures in children treated with spica cast. Clin Orthop 1997;(338):74–8.

48. Hedequist DJ, Sink E. Technical aspects of bridge plating for pediatric femur fractures. J Orthop Trauma 2005;19:276–9.

49. Kanlic EM, Anglen JO, Smith DG, et al. Advantages of submuscular bridge plating for complex pediatric femur fractures. Clin Orthop Relat Res 2004;(426):244–51.

50. Ramseier L, Bhaskar A, Cole W, et al. Treatment of open femur fractures in children: comparison between external fixator and intramedullary nailing. J Pediatr Orthop 2007;27:748–50.

51. Allison P, Dahan-Oliel N, Jando VT, et al. Open fractures of the femur in children: analysis of various treatment methods. J Child Orthop 2011;5(2):101–8.

52. Barlas K, Beg H. Flexible intramedullary nailing versus external fixation of paediatric femoral fractures. Acta Orthop Belg 2006;72(2):159–63.

53. Bar-On E, Sagiv S, Porat S. External fixation or flexible intramedullary nailing for femoral shaft fractures in children. A prospective, randomised study. J Bone Joint Surg Br 1997;79(6):975–8.

54. Bartlett CS 3rd, Weiner LS, Yang EC. Treatment of type II and type III open tibia fractures in children. J Orthop Trauma 1997;11:357–62.

55. Myers SH, Spiegel D, Flynn JM. External fixation of high-energy tibia fractures. J Pediatr Orthop 2007; 27(5):537–9.

56. Skaggs DL, Leet AI, Money MD, et al. Secondary fractures associated with external fixation in pediatric femur fractures. J Pediatr Orthop 1999;19:582–6.

57. Srivastava AK, Mehlman CT, Wall EJ, et al. Elastic stable intramedullary nailing of tibial shaft fractures in children. J Pediatr Orthop 2008;28:152–8.

58. Kubiak EN, Egol KA, Scher D, et al. Operative treatment of tibial fractures in children: are elastic stable intramedullary nails an improvement over external fixation? J Bone Joint Surg Am 2005;87:1761–8.

59. Li Y, Stabile KJ, Shilt JS. Biomechanical analysis of titanium elastic nail fixation in a pediatric femur fracture model. J Pediatr Orthop 2008;28(8):874–8.

60. Özkul E, Gem M, Arslan H, et al. Minimally invasive plate osteosynthesis in open pediatric tibial fractures. J Pediatr Orthop 2015. [Epub ahead of print].

61. Jones BG, Duncan RD. Open tibial fractures in children under 13 years of age—10 years experience. Injury 2003;34:776–80.

62. Buckley SL, Smith G, Sponseller PD, et al. Open fractures of the tibia in children. J Bone Joint Surg Am 1990;72:1462–9.

63. Mosheiff R, Suchar A, Porat S, et al. The "crushed open pelvis" in children. Injury 1999;30(Suppl 2): B14–8.

64. Nugent N, Lynch JB, O'Shaughnessy M, et al. Lawnmower injuries in children. Eur J Emerg Med 2006;13(5):286–9.

65. Erdmann D, Lee B, Roberts CD, et al. Management of lawnmower injuries to the lower extremity in children and adolescents. Ann Plast Surg 2000;45: 595–600.

66. Seymour N. Juxta-epiphysial fracture of the terminal phalanx of the finger. J Bone Joint Surg Br 1966;48:347.

67. Kensinger DR, Guille JT, Horn BD, et al. The stubbed great toe: importance of early recognition and treatment of open fractures of the distal phalanx. J Pediatr Orthop 2001;21(1):31–4.

68. Krusche-Mandl I, Kottstorfer J, Thalhammer G, et al. Seymour fractures: retrospective analysis and therapeutic considerations. J Hand Surg Am 2013;38(2):258–64.

69. Iobst CA, Tidwell MA, King WF. Nonoperative management of pediatric type I open fractures. J Pediatr Orthop 2005;25:513–7.

70. Doak J, Ferrick M. Nonoperative management of pediatric grade 1 open fractures with less than a 24-hour admission. J Pediatr Orthop 2009;29: 49–51.

71. Bazzi AA, Brooks JT, Jain A, et al. Is nonoperative treatment of pediatric type I open fractures safe and effective? J Child Orthop 2014;8(6):467–71.

72. Lewallen RP, Peterson HA. Nonunion of long bone fractures in children: a review of 30 cases. J Pediatr Orthop 1985;5(2):135–42.

73. Hope PG, Cole WG. Open fractures of the tibia in children. J Bone Joint Surg Br 1992;74:546–53.

74. Liow RY, Montgomery RJ. Treatment of established and anticipated nonunion of the tibia in childhood. J Pediatr Orthop 2002;22:754–60.

75. Arslan H, Subaşý M, Kesemenli C, et al. Occurrence and treatment of nonunion in long bone fractures in children. Arch Orthop Trauma Surg 2002;122: 494–8.

76. Schmittenbecher PP, Fitze G, Gödeke J, et al. Delayed healing of forearm shaft fractures in children after intramedullary nailing. J Pediatr Orthop 2008;28(3):303–6.

77. Mesko JW, DeRosa GP, Lindseth RE. Segmental femur loss in children. J Pediatr Orthop 1985;5(4): 471–4.

Compartment Syndrome in Children

Pooya Hosseinzadeh, MD[a],*, Christopher B. Hayes, MD[b]

KEYWORDS

- Compartment syndrome • Intracompartmental pressure • Fasciotomy • Volkman ischemic contracture • Near-infrared spectroscopy

KEY POINTS

- Increased analgesic needs is the first sign of compartment syndrome in children.
- Children with supracondylar humerus fractures, floating elbow injuries, and tibial shaft fractures are at high risk for compartment syndrome.
- Excellent outcome can occur with a timely diagnosis.

INTRODUCTION

Compartment syndrome is one of the true orthopedic emergencies. Regardless of the cause, the combination of rapid influx of fluid into a closed fascial compartment causes elevated intracompartmental pressure. Rising tissue pressure causes decreasing perfusion pressure and ultimately muscle and nerve ischemia. Prolonged ischemia can result in long-term morbidity due to the irreversible damage to muscles, nerves, blood vessels, and skin. Identifying at-risk patients, prompt diagnosis, and treatment are of significant importance. Most cases of compartment syndrome are caused by fractures. Soft tissue injuries in the absence of fractures (especially in children with bleeding disorders) can also lead to compartment syndrome.

Compartment syndrome is a clinical diagnosis, and patient-reported symptoms play a crucial role in recognition of a developing compartment syndrome. Young children cannot properly communicate pain and paresthesia, which can potentially impact the ability of the physician to make the diagnosis of compartment syndrome in a timely fashion. These patients may be admitted to pediatric floors that routinely do not care for orthopedic patients and whose staff may not be familiar with signs and symptoms of increased intracompartmental pressures. Physicians and other health care professionals (nurses, physician assistants, and others) taking care of children should be aware of unique features of compartment syndrome in children and should be able to identify at-risk patients that benefit from close monitoring.

The best approach to compartment syndrome relies on constant vigilance and decisive action to avert irreversible tissue damage. In addition, from a medicolegal standpoint, early diagnosis is very important. Only 44% of cases of compartment syndrome are closed in favor of treating physician compared with 75% of cases in other orthopedic malpractice claims.[1,2]

CLASSIFICATION

Compartment syndrome can be classified into the following types.

Acute Compartment Syndrome

Acute compartment syndrome is the most common form of compartment syndrome caused by an acute increase in the intracompartmental pressure, causing tissue ischemia. Currently,

Conflict of Interest: No conflicts of interest to disclose.
[a] Department of Orthopedics, Herbert Wertheim College of Medicine, Florida International University, Baptist Children's Hospital, 8740 North Kendall Drive, Suite 115, Miami, FL 33176, USA; [b] Department of Orthopedics, University of Kentucky, 740 South Limestone, Room J-111, Lexington, KY 40536, USA
* Corresponding author.
E-mail address: pooyah@baptisthealth.net

Orthop Clin N Am 47 (2016) 579–587
http://dx.doi.org/10.1016/j.ocl.2016.02.004

acute compartment syndrome of the leg is the most commonly seen scenario in children.

Exercise-induced Compartment Syndrome

Exercised-induced compartment syndrome is caused by reversible tissue ischemia caused by noncomplaint fascial compartment that cannot accommodate muscle expansion in exercise. It has been reported in both upper and lower extremities.

Neonatal Compartment Syndrome

Neonatal compartment syndrome is a rare form of compartment syndrome caused potentially by birth trauma and low perfusion of the extremities. It has only been reported in the upper extremity.

Volkmann Ischemic Contracture

Volkmann ischemic contracture is the consequence of prolonged ischemia and irreversible tissue loss, which is most commonly associated with supracondylar humerus fractures in children.

PATHOPHYSIOLOGY

Acute compartment syndrome can be caused by either fracture or reperfusion injury with unique pathophysiology regarding both causes. This article focuses on compartment syndrome relating to fracture. Acute compartment syndrome is caused by either bleeding or edema within a closed osseofascial compartment, leading to a reduction in perfusion of the contained muscles and nerves. Most studies of compartment syndrome have been undertaken as retrospective reviews of adult trauma patients or induced within animal models.

Early studies sought to determine the pathophysiology of compartment syndrome in hopes of determining the critical thresholds before it must be addressed. The underlying pathogenesis, however, has remained elusive, and still some controversy exists as to the underlying cause. Initially, 3 main theories persisted. Some have hypothesized its origin is from venous obstruction.[3–5] Others thought the basic problem was that of diminished arterial inflow.[6,7] Finally, others thought the root cause to be obstruction of inflow due to arterial spasm.[8,9] Recently, the underlying root cause of compartment syndrome was elucidated with the use of a novel animal system using hamster-striated muscle and in vivo fluorescence microscopy. The main determinant of diminished compartment perfusion was determined to be due to increasing intracompartmental pressure causing

venular compression. This compression thereby causes a diminution in the arteriovenous pressure gradient, thus decreasing blood flow and perfusion to the compartmental skeletal muscle and nervous tissue.[10] Normal cellular metabolism requires an oxygen tension of at least 5 to 7 mm Hg to sustain life. Once blood flow decreases and oxygen is used up, the oxygen tension quickly decreases, resulting in ischemia, and normal cellular metabolism can no longer be sustained.

As a result of ischemia, muscle and nerve tissue quickly lose their function. Nerve demonstrates the most sensitivity to initial ischemia with functional abnormalities, including paresthesia and hypoesthesia within 30 minutes of ischemic onset. However, irreversible functional loss does not occur until after 12 to 24 hours of continued ischemia.[11–14] Muscle, on the other hand, demonstrates prolonged functional capacity for at least 2 to 4 hours following onset of ischemia; however, muscle begins to exhibit irreversible functional loss beginning at 4 hours after ischemic onset.[13,15,16] Because of these landmark studies, the authors have been able to determine optimal time to treatment for this limb- and sometimes life-threatening complication.

DIAGNOSIS

Compartment syndrome is a clinical diagnosis, and patient-reported symptoms play a crucial role in the recognition of a developing compartment syndrome. Identifying an evolving compartment syndrome in a young child is difficult because of the child's limited ability to properly communicate and the potential anxiety during examination. Orthopedic surgeons have been trained for generations to look for the 5 Ps (pain, paresthesia, paralysis, pallor, and pulselessness) associated with compartment syndrome. Pain out of proportion and pain with passive stretch are known as the first signs of an evolving compartment syndrome. Examining an anxious young child is difficult, and documenting the amount of pain may not be practical in children.

In a retrospective report of 33 children diagnosed with compartment syndrome at Boston Children's Hospital, Bae and colleagues[17] reported the traditional 5 Ps to be relatively unreliable in children. They reported that increasing analgesic need was found on average 7 hours before change in the vascular status and was a more sensitive indicator of compartment syndrome in children. They recommended that children at risk for compartment syndrome be monitored for the 3 As (increasing analgesic requirement, anxiety, and agitation) (Table 1).[18]

Measurement of compartment pressure can be helpful in decision-making in certain clinical scenarios. Compartment pressure measurement in an obtunded child or a child with mental disability can help confirm or rule out the diagnosis.

Normal resting leg compartment pressures in children are reported to be higher compared with adults. Staudt and colleagues[19] reported compartment pressure measurements in 4 lower leg compartments in 20 healthy children and compared that with 20 healthy adults using the same technique. Measured compartment pressures in children in 4 leg compartments varied between 13.3 mm Hg and 16.6 mm Hg, and compartment pressure measurements in adults varied between 5.2 mm Hg and 9.7 mm Hg, which indicates a higher normal resting pressure in lower leg compartments in children. The clinical relevance of this finding is not yet defined.

Compartment pressures are reported to be highest within 5 cm of the fracture site and should be measured close to fracture site when clinically indicated.[20] The pressure threshold that would require fasciotomy is debatable. Intracompartmental pressures of 30 to 45 mm Hg or measurements less than 30 mm Hg of diastolic blood pressure (ΔP = diastolic blood pressure − compartment pressure) are recommended by some investigators as the cutoff points.[21–24] These cutoff values cannot be used as reliably in children because of the differences in resting normal compartment pressures between children and adults. Compartment pressure measurement is painful and can be difficult in an agitated and awake child. The utility of near-infrared spectroscopy in the diagnosis of increased compartment pressure has been reported.[25,26] This method uses differential light absorption properties of oxygenated hemoglobin to measure tissue ischemia similar to the method used in pulse oximetry. Near-infrared spectroscopy is able to sample deeper tissue (3 cm below the skin level) than pulse oximetry. In a report of near-infrared spectroscopy findings of 14 adults with acute compartment syndrome, Shuler and colleagues[25] reported that lower tissue oxygenation levels correlated with increased intracompartmental pressures but were not able to define a cutoff value for which measurements would indicate significant tissue ischemia. The use of near-infrared spectroscopy for diagnosis of compartment syndrome in children is also recently reported.[26]

Compartment syndrome remains a clinical diagnosis. Clinicians should be proactive in those scenarios where increased risk exists. Informing family and staff about the signs and symptoms of this syndrome and close monitoring of analgesic use are critical. Compartment pressure measurement is used when diagnosis is not clear, but these values should be interpreted with caution.

CHILDREN AT HIGH RISK FOR ACUTE COMPARTMENT SYNDROME AFTER TRAUMA

Children with certain injuries are at high risk for compartment syndrome. These injuries are discussed in detail later.

Supracondylar Humerus Fracture

Compartment syndrome is reported to develop in 0.1% to 0.3% of children with supracondylar humerus fractures.[27,28] Volar compartment of the forearm is the most common affected compartment in this group of patients. Elbow flexion more than 90° in a cast and vascular injury put these children at increased risk of compartment syndrome. In a report of 9 cases of compartment syndrome in the volar compartment of the forearm after supracondylar humerus fractures, 8 of 9 cases were attributed to elbow flexion beyond 90° after closed reduction.[29] Highest compartment pressures after supracondylar humerus fractures are reported in the deep volar compartment of the forearm close to the fracture site. Significant increase in compartment pressures was also reported with elbow flexion beyond 90°.[27]

Choi and colleagues[30] reported 2 cases of compartment syndrome in 9 patients with supracondylar humerus fractures who presented without a pulse and without adequate hand

Table 1	
Signs of compartment syndrome (5 Ps and 3 As)	
5 Ps	**3 As**
Pain	Increased Analgesic
Paresthesia	requirement
Pallor	Anxiety
Paralysis	Agitation
Pulselessness	

Data from Bae DS, Kadiyala RK, Waters PM. Acute compartment syndrome in children: contemporary diagnosis, treatment, and outcome. J Pediatr Orthop 2001;21(5):680–8; and Noonan KJ, McCarthy JJ. Compartment syndrome in the pediatric patient. J Pediatr Orthop 2010;30(Suppl 2):96–101.

perfusion. No cases of compartment syndrome were seen in 24 children who presented with pulseless but well perfused hand in the same case series.

Several recent reports have shown that a delay of 8 to 12 hours in the treatment of Gartland type 2 and type 3 supracondylar humerus fractures does not increase the rate of compartment syndrome.[31–34] These studies did not recommend treatment delays in patients who present without a radial pulse or with a neurologic deficit. A recent multicenter case series reported 11 cases of acute compartment syndrome in patients who initially presented with a low-energy supracondylar humerus fracture and intact radial pulse. All these patients presented with severe swelling and had a mean delay of 22 hours (6–64 hours) before surgery.[28] Diagnosis of acute compartment syndrome can be challenging in patients with supracondylar humerus fractures and median nerve palsy due to decreased pain sensation caused by the nerve palsy. Based on the above-mentioned reports, the authors do not recommend delayed treatment of children with supracondylar humerus fracture who present with a neurologic deficit or absent pulse and recommend close monitoring of patients with severe swelling.

Although volar compartment of the forearm is mostly affected in cases of compartment syndrome seen in patients with supracondylar humerus fractures, compartment syndrome of the mobile wad, anterior arm compartment, and posterior arm compartment are also reported in the literature.[35,36]

Floating Elbow
Children with ipsilateral displaced distal humerus and forearm fractures are reported to be at high risk for compartment syndrome. Blakemore and colleagues[37] reported 3 cases of acute compartment syndrome among 9 patients (33%) who presented with displaced extension-type supracondylar humerus and displaced ipsilateral forearm fractures. A report of 16 children who presented with displaced ipsilateral distal humerus and forearm fractures to Boston Children's Hospital showed 2 cases of acute compartment syndrome and 4 cases of impending compartment syndrome among 10 patients who were treated by closed reduction and circumferential casting for forearm fractures. No signs of compartment syndrome were reported in the 6 patients who were treated by K-wire fixation of both distal humerus and forearm fractures.[38] Based on the above-mentioned reports, the authors do not

recommend circumferential casting to treat displaced forearm fractures in children presenting with floating elbow injuries.

In a recent report of the largest series of children with floating elbow injuries, Muchow and colleagues[39] did not report any cases of compartment syndrome among 150 children who presented with ipsilateral distal humerus and forearm fractures. They reported a higher rate of neurologic deficit at presentation among children with floating elbow injuries when compared with children with isolated distal humerus fractures.

Forearm Fractures
Children with fractures of the radius and ulnar shaft can develop acute compartment syndrome. Haasbeek and Cole[40] reported 5 cases of acute compartment syndrome among 46 children (11%) with open forearm fractures. In a report of cases of compartment syndrome after intramedullary nailing of forearm fractures in children, Yuan and colleagues[41] reported 3 cases of compartment syndrome (6%) among 50 patients with open forearm fractures and 3 cases of compartment syndrome among 30 patients with closed forearm fractures treated by closed reduction and intramedullary nailing. In this study, the increased intraoperative time was associated with the increased risk of developing postoperative compartment syndrome. The investigators discussed the prolonged closed manipulation of forearm fractures before intramedullary nailing as a risk factor for the development of postoperative compartment syndrome. In this study, no cases of compartment syndrome were reported among 205 forearm fractures treated by closed reduction and casting.

Flynn and colleagues[42] reported 2 cases of acute compartment syndrome among 30 patients treated with intramedullary nailing within 24 hours of injury and did not report any cases of compartment syndrome in 73 patients treated with intramedullary nailing after 24 hours of the injury. In this study, intramedullary nailing within the first 24 hours from the injury was reported as a risk factor for developing compartment syndrome in children with radius and ulna fractures.

Blackman and colleagues[43] reported 3 cases of acute compartment syndrome among 39 patients (7.7%) with open forearm fractures and did not report any cases of compartment syndrome in 74 children with closed forearm fractures treated operatively. In this case series, a small incision was made to facilitate reduction in 38 of 74 patients with closed fractures (51.4%) in order to decrease the closed manipulation time and operative time. The rate of compartment syndrome after intramedullary nailing of closed forearm fractures in this series is lower than other reports in the literature, which could be due to the decreased closed manipulation and operative time.

Based on the current data in the literature, children with open forearm fractures and children with forearm fractures treated by closed reduction and intramedullary nailing are at increased risk of developing acute compartment syndrome especially if intramedullary nailing is performed within 24 hours of the injury and/or if prolonged closed manipulation of the fracture is performed during surgery. The authors recommend close monitoring of all children treated operatively for forearm fractures, especially children who have the above-mentioned risk factors. Prolonged closed manipulation before intramedullary nailing is not recommended because of the potential increased risk of compartment syndrome.

Tibia Fractures

Currently, the most common scenario for compartment syndrome in children is the acute compartment syndrome of the leg. Children with tibia fractures, especially those caused by motor vehicle accidents, are at risk for developing compartment syndrome. In one report, compartment syndrome is reported in 4 of 92 children (4%) with open tibia fractures.[44]

Children with tibial tubercle fractures are at increased risk of developing compartment syndrome because of the concomitant vascular injury seen with this fracture (injury to anterior tibial recurrent artery). In one report, compartment syndrome or vascular compromise was seen in 4 of 40 patients with tibial tubercle fractures.[45]

Flynn and colleagues[46] reported 43 cases of acute compartment syndrome of the leg in 42 skeletally immature children from 2 pediatric trauma centers. Thirty-five (83%) of the 42 cases were seen in children with tibia and fibula fractures caused by motor vehicle accidents. Average reported time from injury to fasciotomy was 20.5 hours (3.9–118 hours) in this study. This study shows a potential slow development and delayed presentation or delayed diagnosis of acute compartment syndrome of the leg in children.

In a recent report from Boston Children's Hospital, 25 cases of acute compartment syndrome were reported among 216 patients (11.6%) with tibia fractures.[47] Acute compartment syndrome was diagnosed clinically or by compartment pressure measurements in this study. The investigators reported that children with motor vehicle accidents and children older than 14 are at higher risk for acute compartment syndrome after tibia fractures. In this study, compartment syndrome developed in 12 (48%) of 25 children older than 14 years of age who sustained a motor vehicle accident. The rate of compartment syndrome after tibia fractures reported in this study is higher than previously reported rates in the literature, which could be due to the frequent use of compartment pressure measurements for the diagnosis of compartment syndrome in this study.

Close monitoring of children with high-energy tibial shaft fractures and children with tibial tubercle fractures for signs of compartment syndrome is recommended.

Mubarak[48] reported 6 patients with distal tibial physeal fractures who presented with severe pain and swelling of the ankle, hypoesthesia in the first web space, weakness of the extensor hallucis longus and the extensor digitorum communis muscles, and pain with passive flexion of the toes. Compartment pressure measurements showed measurements more than 40 mm Hg beneath the extensor retinaculum and less than 20 mm Hg in the anterior compartment in all 6 patients. Prompt relief of the pain and improved sensation and strength within 24 hours of the release of the superior extensor retinaculum and fracture stabilization were reported in all of these patients. This study reported a unique type of increased intracompartmental pressure in children with distal tibia fractures that would benefit from fascial release.

Femur Fractures

Compartment syndrome after femur fractures is not common and may be related to casting techniques. Compartment syndrome and Volkmann contracture are reported after 90 of 90 spica casting of femur fractures in children. In one report, 9 cases of calf compartment syndrome and Volkmann contracture were reported in children with femur fractures treated in 90 of 90 spica casts.[49] One specific technique while applying the cast (applying the short leg cast first and applying traction through the short leg cast) was attributed to this complication by the investigators. This technique must be avoided when applying long leg casts and spica casts in children. The investigators recommended an alternative method of applying spica casts, which is beyond the scope of this review.

Miscellaneous and Nontraumatic Causes of Compartment Syndrome

Neonatal compartment syndrome is very rare, and the diagnosis is often missed. It is thought to be caused by a combination of low neonatal blood pressure and birth trauma.[50] Ragland and colleagues[51] reported 24 cases of neonatal compartment syndrome. In their series, the diagnosis was made within 24 hours in only 1 patient, which resulted in good clinical outcome.[18] They described a "sentinel skin lesion" (Fig. 1) on the forearm of these patients as the sign of neonatal compartment syndrome. High clinical suspicion is the key to early diagnosis and treatment of this rare abnormality.

Medical problems causing intracompartmental bleeding (liver and renal failure, leukemia, coagulopathy) could potentially cause acute compartment syndrome.[52,53] Correction of the coagulation defect may take priority over surgical treatment in these cases, although the decision should be made on a case-by-case basis.[52]

Snake bites can cause compartment syndrome in children. Successful use of antivenin in prevention of surgical treatment is reported by Shaw and Hosalkar.[54] Sixteen of 19 patients with rattlesnake bites were treated with antivenin and did not require surgical treatment. In their report, 2 patients had limited surgical debridement and only one patient underwent fasciotomy.[54]

Prasarn and colleagues[2] reported 12 cases of acute compartment syndrome of the upper extremity in children without the evidence of obvious fractures. Ten of these 12 patients were managed in the intensive care unit and had an obtunded sensorium. The cause in 7 of

12 cases (58%) was iatrogenic (intravenous infiltration, retained phlebotomy tourniquet). Four amputations were performed on the affected extremities in this series. Diagnosis of compartment syndrome in an obtunded patient can be very challenging. Compartment pressure measurements would be beneficial in early diagnosis and treatment of an obtunded patient who is at risk for developing compartment syndrome.

TREATMENT

The most effective treatment of compartment syndrome is the anticipation of high-risk situations and avoidance of a critical increase in the compartment pressure. External sources of compression such as circumferential dressings should be split and casts bivalved prophylactically in high-risk patients, or at the onset of increasing pain. Moreover, the vascular input to the traumatized area should be optimized to maintain perfusion pressure. The injured limb should only be elevated to the level of the heart, and blood pressure should be supported if medically possible. If the diagnosis of compartment syndrome is made, emergent fasciotomy and decompression are indicated. Definitive treatment of the cause of compartment syndrome should also be kept in mind while planning fasciotomy. Treatment of clotting deficiency in cases caused by excessive bleeding, fracture fixation, and vascular repair may be indicated while performing fasciotomy and decompression.

In cases of compartment syndrome of the forearm, a volar incision is used to decompress superficial and deep compartments as well as the carpal tunnel. Dorsal decompression may be needed if the mobile wad and dorsal compartments are involved.

In leg compartment syndrome, all 4 compartments (anterior, lateral, superficial, and deep posterior) should be fully decompressed. This depression can be achieved with either a 2-incision (medial and anterolateral) or 1-incision (lateral) technique.

Delayed primary skin closure and split thickness skin grafting are the common methods used for closure. Vacuum-assisted closure can be used before final closure.[18,55]

OUTCOMES

A recent study by Flynn and colleagues[46] reported the outcome of 43 cases of acute compartment syndrome of the leg in children from 2 pediatric trauma centers. Average time

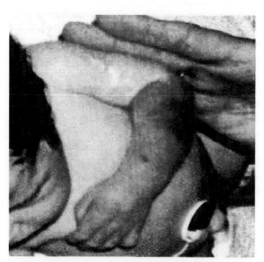

Fig. 1. Skin lesion in neonatal compartment syndrome of the forearm. (*From* Ragland R 3rd, Moukoko D, Ezaki M, et al. Forearm compartment syndrome in the newborn: report of 24 cases. J Hand Surg Am 2005;30(5):999; with permission.)

from injury to fasciotomy was 20.5 hours (3.9–118 hours) in this report. Excellent functional outcome was reported at the time of follow-up. Forty-one of the 43 cases had no sequelae at the time of follow-up. Two patients that lost function in this study had fasciotomies performed more than 80 hours after injury. In this report, despite a long period from injury to surgery, excellent results were reported with fasciotomy, which may suggest an increased potential for recovery in children.

Bae and colleagues[17] reported outcomes of 33 cases of acute compartment syndrome of the upper and the lower extremity treated at Boston Children's Hospital. All cases were treated with fasciotomy and the average follow-up was 26.1 months. Full functional recovery was achieved in 30 of 33 cases (91%) by an average of 2.5 months from surgery.

SUMMARY

Compartment syndrome is a complication that should be anticipated in high-risk patients and actively avoided if possible. However, in those cases when the compartment pressure exceeds the perfusion pressure, irreversible damage can occur. An increase in analgesic needs is often the first sign of compartment syndrome in children, and analgesic use should be monitored closely in children who are at high risk for developing compartment syndrome. Compartment syndrome continues to be a clinical diagnosis, and compartment pressure measurement should only be performed as a confirmatory test in noncommunicative patients or when the diagnosis is not clear. Children with supracondylar humerus fractures, forearm fractures treated operatively, tibial shaft fractures, tibial tubercle fractures, and medical risk factors for coagulopathy are at increased risk and should be monitored closely. When diagnosed and treated promptly, good long-term results can be expected.

REFERENCES

1. Bhattacharyya T, Vrahas MS. The medical-legal aspects of compartment syndrome. J Bone Joint Surg Am 2004;86A(4):864–8.
2. Prasarn ML, Ouellette EA, Livingstone A, et al. Acute pediatric upper extremity compartment syndrome in the absence of fracture. J Pediatr Orthop 2009;29(3):263–8.
3. Leach RE, Hammond G, Stryker WS. Anterior tibial compartment syndrome. Acute and chronic. J Bone Joint Surg Am 1967;49(3):451–62.
4. Paton DF. The pathogenesis of anterior tibial syndrome. An illustrative case. J Bone Joint Surg Br 1968;50(2):383–5.
5. Rorabeck CH, Macnab I. The pathophysiology of the anterior tibial compartmental syndrome. Clin Orthop Relat Res 1975;(113):52–7.
6. Freedman BJ, Knowles CH. Anterior tibial syndrome due to arterial embolism and thrombosis; ischaemic necrosis of the anterior crural muscles. Br Med J 1959;2(5147):270–5.
7. Horn CE. Acute ischemia of the anterior tibial muscle and the long extensor muscles of the toes. J Bone Joint Surg 1945;27(4):615–22.
8. Benjamin A. The relief of traumatic arterial spasm in threatened Volkmann's ischaemic contracture. J Bone Joint Surg Br 1957;39B(4):711–3.
9. Eaton RG, Green WT. Epimysiotomy and fasciotomy in the treatment of Volkmann's ischemic contracture. Orthop Clin North Am 1972;3(1):175–86.
10. Vollmar B, Westermann S, Menger MD. Microvascular response to compartment syndrome-like external pressure elevation: an in vivo fluorescence microscopic study in the hamster striated muscle. J Trauma 1999;46(1):91–6.
11. Bowden RE, Gutmann E. The fate of voluntary muscle after vascular injury in man. J Bone Joint Surg Br 1949;31B(3):356–68.
12. Holmes W, Highet WB, Seddon HJ. Ischaemic nerve lesions occurring in Volkmann's contracture. Br J Surg 1944;32(126):259–75.
13. Malan E, Tattoni G. Physio- and anatomo-pathology of acute ischemia of the extremities. J Cardiovasc Surg (Torino) 1963;4:212–25.
14. Parkes AR. Traumatic ischaemia of peripheral nerves–with some observations on Volkmann's ischaemic contracture. Br J Surg 1945;32(127):403–14.
15. Harman JW, Gwinn RP. The recovery of skeletal muscle fibers from acute ischemia as determined by histologic and chemical methods. Am J Pathol 1949;25(4):741–55.
16. Scully RE, Shannon JM, Dickersin GR. Factors involved in recovery from experimental skeletal muscle ischemia produced in dogs: I. Histologic and histochemical pattern of ischemic muscle. Am J Pathol 1961;39(6):721–37.
17. Bae DS, Kadiyala RK, Waters PM. Acute compartment syndrome in children: contemporary diagnosis, treatment, and outcome. J Pediatr Orthop 2001;21(5):680–8.
18. Noonan KJ, McCarthy JJ. Compartment syndrome in the pediatric patient. J Pediatr Orthop 2010;30(Suppl 2):96–101.
19. Staudt JM, Smeulders MJ, van der Horst CM. Normal compartment pressures of the lower leg in children. J Bone Joint Surg Br 2008;90(2):215–9.

20. Heckman MM, Whitesides TE Jr, Grewe SR, et al. Compartment pressure in association with closed tibial fractures. The relationship between tissue pressure, compartment, and the distance from the site of the fracture. J Bone Joint Surg Am 1994;76(9):1285–92.

21. Hargens AR, Schmidt DA, Evans KL, et al. Quantitation of skeletal-muscle necrosis in a model compartment syndrome. J Bone Joint Surg Am 1981;63(4):631–6.

22. Heppenstall RB, Sapega AA, Scott R, et al. The compartment syndrome. An experimental and clinical study of muscular energy metabolism using phosphorus nuclear magnetic resonance spectroscopy. Clin Orthop Relat Res 1988;(226):138–55.

23. McQueen MM, Court-Brown CM. Compartment monitoring in tibial fractures. The pressure threshold for decompression. J Bone Joint Surg Br 1996;78(1):99–104.

24. Rorabeck CH. The treatment of compartment syndromes of the leg. J Bone Joint Surg Br 1984; 66(1):93–7.

25. Shuler MS, Reisman WM, Kinsey TL, et al. Correlation between muscle oxygenation and compartment pressures in acute compartment syndrome of the leg. J Bone Joint Surg Am 2010;92(4): 863–70.

26. Tobias JD, Hoernschemeyer DG. Near-infrared spectroscopy identifies compartment syndrome in an infant. J Pediatr Orthop 2007;27(3):311–3.

27. Battaglia TC, Armstrong DG, Schwend RM. Factors affecting forearm compartment pressures in children with supracondylar fractures of the humerus. J Pediatr Orthop 2002;22(4):431–9.

28. Ramachandran M, Skaggs DL, Crawford HA, et al. Delaying treatment of supracondylar fractures in children: has the pendulum swung too far? J Bone Joint Surg Br 2008;90(9):1228–33.

29. Mubarak SJ, Carroll NC. Volkmann's contracture in children: aetiology and prevention. J Bone Joint Surg Br 1979;61B(3):285–93.

30. Choi PD, Melikian R, Skaggs DL. Risk factors for vascular repair and compartment syndrome in the pulseless supracondylar humerus fracture in children. J Pediatr Orthop 2010;30(1):50–6.

31. Gupta N, Kay RM, Leitch K, et al. Effect of surgical delay on perioperative complications and need for open reduction in supracondylar humerus fractures in children. J Pediatr Orthop 2004;24(3):245–8.

32. Iyengar SR, Hoffinger SA, Townsend DR. Early versus delayed reduction and pinning of type III displaced supracondylar fractures of the humerus in children: a comparative study. J Orthop Trauma 1999;13(1):51–5.

33. Leet AI, Frisancho J, Ebramzadeh E. Delayed treatment of type 3 supracondylar humerus fractures in children. J Pediatr Orthop 2002;22(2):203–7.

34. Mehlman CT, Strub WM, Roy DR, et al. The effect of surgical timing on the perioperative complications of treatment of supracondylar humeral fractures in children. J Bone Joint Surg Am 2001; 83A(3):323–7.

35. Diesselhorst MM, Deck JW, Davey JP. Compartment syndrome of the upper arm after closed reduction and percutaneous pinning of a supracondylar humerus fracture. J Pediatr Orthop 2014;34(2): e1–4.

36. Mai MC, Beck R, Gabriel K, et al. Posterior arm compartment syndrome after a combined supracondylar humeral and capitellar fractures in an adolescent: a case report. J Pediatr Orthop 2011; 31(3):e16–9.

37. Blakemore LC, Cooperman DR, Thompson GH, et al. Compartment syndrome in ipsilateral humerus and forearm fractures in children. Clin Orthop Relat Res 2000;(376):32–8.

38. Ring D, Waters PM, Hotchkiss RN, et al. Pediatric floating elbow. J Pediatr Orthop 2001;21(4):456–9.

39. Muchow RD, Riccio AI, Garg S, et al. Neurological and vascular injury associated with supracondylar humerus fractures and ipsilateral forearm fractures in children. J Pediatr Orthop 2015;35(2):121–5.

40. Haasbeek JF, Cole WG. Open fractures of the arm in children. J Bone Joint Surg Br 1995;77(4):576–81.

41. Yuan PS, Pring ME, Gaynor TP, et al. Compartment syndrome following intramedullary fixation of pediatric forearm fractures. J Pediatr Orthop 2004;24(4): 370–5.

42. Flynn JM, Jones KJ, Garner MR, et al. Eleven years experience in the operative management of pediatric forearm fractures. J Pediatr Orthop 2010; 30(4):313–9.

43. Blackman AJ, Wall LB, Keeler KA, et al. Acute compartment syndrome after intramedullary nailing of isolated radius and ulna fractures in children. J Pediatr Orthop 2014;34(1):50–4.

44. Hope PG, Cole WG. Open fractures of the tibia in children. J Bone Joint Surg Br 1992;74(4):546–53.

45. Pandya NK, Edmonds EW, Roocroft JH, et al. Tibial tubercle fractures: complications, classification, and the need for intra-articular assessment. J Pediatr Orthop 2012;32(8):749–59.

46. Flynn JM, Bashyal RK, Yeger-McKeever M, et al. Acute traumatic compartment syndrome of the leg in children: diagnosis and outcome. J Bone Joint Surg Am 2011;93(10):937–41.

47. Shore BJ, Glotzbecker MP, Zurakowski D, et al. Acute compartment syndrome in children and teenagers with tibial shaft fractures: incidence and multivariable risk factors. J Orthop Trauma 2013; 27(11):616–21.

48. Mubarak SJ. Extensor retinaculum syndrome of the ankle after injury to the distal tibial physis. J Bone Joint Surg Br 2002;84(1):11–4.

49. Mubarak SJ, Frick S, Sink E, et al. Volkmann contracture and compartment syndromes after femur fractures in children treated with 90/90 spica casts. J Pediatr Orthop 2006;26(5):567–72.

50. Macer GA Jr. Forearm compartment syndrome in the newborn. J Hand Surg Am 2006;31(9):1550.

51. Ragland R 3rd, Moukoko D, Ezaki M, et al. Forearm compartment syndrome in the newborn: report of 24 cases. J Hand Surg Am 2005;30(5): 997–1003.

52. Alioglu B, Avci Z, Baskin E, et al. Successful use of recombinant factor VIIa (NovoSeven) in children

with compartment syndrome: two case reports. J Pediatr Orthop 2006;26(6):815–7.

53. Lee DK, Jeong WK, Lee DH, et al. Multiple compartment syndrome in a pediatric patient with CML. J Pediatr Orthop 2011;31(8):889–92.

54. Shaw BA, Hosalkar HS. Rattlesnake bites in children: antivenin treatment and surgical indications. J Bone Joint Surg Am 2002;84A(9):1624–9.

55. Yang CC, Chang DS, Webb LX. Vacuum-assisted closure for fasciotomy wounds following compartment syndrome of the leg. J Surg Orthop Adv 2006;15(1):19–23.

Upper Extremity

Acute Ischemia of the Upper Extremity

William C. Pederson, MD

KEYWORDS

- Vascular • Ischemia • Hand • Trauma • Thrombosis

KEY POINTS

- Open vascular injury should be managed with exploration.
- Ulnar and radial artery thrombosis in the hand may be managed conservatively in some patients.
- Subclavian artery and vein thrombosis in high-level athletes often requires surgery, but the patient can usually return to sports.

Acute ischemia in the upper extremity is an uncommon occurrence in orthopedic trauma but can pose significant problems if it occurs. An ischemic hand is most common after open trauma, and is often the result of cutting injuries or firearms; however, it can present after a closed injury. A review of a large series of civilian traumatic vascular injuries revealed that 18% occurred in the upper extremity.[1] Significant arterial injury with ischemia of the hand presents a surgical emergency, and restoring flow to the injured limb usually takes precedence over the management of other injuries. In the large series of civilian vascular injuries mentioned previously, however, with appropriate vascular intervention major and minor amputation rates remain less than 5%.[2]

OPEN TRAUMA

Open injuries to the upper extremity may cause injury to a major arterial structure, which can lead to ischemia of the distal limb. This more commonly occurs in the upper arm with injury to the brachial artery, because injury to either the radial or ulnar artery in the forearm should not lead to ischemia in the hand. Injury to both vessels in the forearm can lead to an ischemic hand, but these injuries are usually amputations or near-amputations. In any event, the vascular injury needs to be addressed in terms of re-establishing flow to the hand before undertaking management of the bony and soft tissue injuries. Muscle only tolerates 4 to 6 hours of warm ischemia,[3] and thus restoring arterial flow quickly to the ischemic limb is paramount.

In general, a patient with an open injury to the upper limb and an ischemic hand requires urgent exploration in the operating room. Physical examination with Doppler examination of pulses in the emergency department, along with appropriate radiographs to evaluate bony trauma is probably all that is necessary in these patients. Although other imaging studies might be helpful, the delay required for performing vascular studies is generally not warranted. The wounds need to be managed regardless, and thus expeditious exploration in the operating room after hemodynamic stabilization of the patient is the proper course of action.

Once the patient is stabilized and is taken to the operating room, flow can be restored temporarily with an arterial shunt. This technique has been proven to be reliable and was used in several patients during recent military conflicts.[4,5] Published studies have shown that shunts can be used to control hemorrhage from vascular injuries and to reperfuse distal tissue. They can also be placed as a temporizing measure until surgeons with expertise in the

---

The author receives royalties from Elsevier as a textbook editor.

Texas Children's Hospital, Baylor College of Medicine, 6701 Fannin, Suite 610, Houston, TX 77030, USA

E-mail addresses: wcpeders@texaschildrens.org; micro1@ix.netcom.com

http://dx.doi.org/10.1016/j.ocl.2016.03.004

area of vascular repair are available, or even left in place to allow perfusion of the limb while the patient is transferred. Studies have shown that the results of placing a shunt temporarily (hours up to a day or more) are the same as performing a vascular repair at the initial exploration.[6] An arterial shunt can be placed while bony fixation is performed, and a definitive repair done once bony stabilization has been achieved.

A Javid-type shunt of the appropriate size is chosen and flushed with heparinized saline. The shunt is place in the vessel ends and held in place with either a special clamp designed for this purpose or an umbilical tape placed around the vessel and clamped down via a piece of red rubber catheter (Fig. 1). In most instances, this shunt is left in place only long enough to allow for bony stabilization, at which time definitive repair of the vascular injury is performed. It has been shown feasible to leave the shunt in for 6 hours or longer[7] if the patient is unstable or needs transfer.

Definitive repair of major arterial injury in the upper extremity can sometimes be performed primarily if the injury is a sharp laceration. In these cases the injured vessel end is trimmed back and the vessel is freed up for a few centimeters by taking down small local side branches (Fig. 2). In most instances of significant trauma with open fracture, however, resection of the injured portion of the vessel and reversed vein grafting is required (Fig. 3). This is done with either the cephalic or basilic veins from the arm or saphenous from the leg. Whichever vein is chosen, it should be reversed to prevent the venous valves from obstructing distal flow.

The basic principle of vascular surgery is proximal and distal control of the injured vessels. In the upper extremity this is usually fairly straightforward because surgery can often start with a tourniquet applied. Regardless, wide exposure of the vessel is necessary to gain appropriate control and place vascular clamps, and thus incisions should be made or extended as necessary to allow for proper visualization. Blind clamping of a bleeding vessel is to be condemned, because it can lead to further trauma and potentially damage uninjured nerves, which increases the morbidity of the injury. If necessary, finger pressure is held on a bleeding vessel while an incision is made proximal to the site of injury over the injured vessel where this can be exposed and controlled. If exposure is very difficult (for example in the axilla), the end of the vessel is identified and a Fogarty balloon catheter of the appropriate size placed in the lumen of the damaged vessel and the balloon inflated. This can occlude flow until better exposure is obtained. Once the vessels are clamped, one should irrigate proximally and distally with heparinized saline to decrease the risk of thrombosis while the clamps are in place. If flow from the proximal vessel is not good one may need to consider using a balloon catheter to remove thrombus before attempting repair. This technique is beyond the scope of this article but is reviewed in standard textbooks on vascular surgery.[8]

Once proximal and distal control is secured, the ends of the vessel should be trimmed back to an uninjured area and the defect between the ends measured. An appropriate length of graft is marked out over the selected vein and this vein is then harvested. The vein is marked so that it can be reversed and brought up to the site of arterial injury. I prefer to perform the proximal anastomosis first, in arteries the size of the brachial artery generally using a 6–0 or 7–0 polypropylene suture, with either an interrupted or continuous suture technique. For the smaller vessels in the forearm I use an 8–0 nylon for repair and generally use an interrupted suturing technique (see Fig. 2D). In the case of severe degloving injuries, repair of

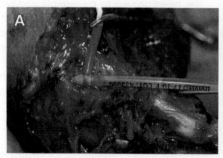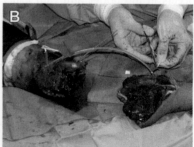

Fig. 1. (A) View of Javid shunt placed on proximal vessel after being flushed with heparinized saline. Note umbilical tape pulled around vessel and held in place with portion of red rubber catheter and clamp. Tourniquet is currently up so there is no flow through the shunt. (B) Shunt connected proximally and distally before tourniquet deflation.

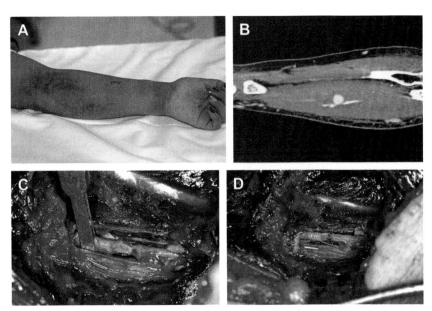

Fig. 2. (A) View of arm of 24-year-old woman who suffered a stab wound to the forearm. This was sutured in an outlying hospital and she presented 8 hours later with a tensely swollen forearm and increasing pain. (B) Computed tomography scan obtained by emergency room shows leak from ulnar artery. (C) View of vessel at time of exploration with incomplete division of ulnar artery. (D) Artery after repair with 8–0 nylon.

venous structures may be required but these in general proceed in a similar manner to arterial repair and/or grafting.

Postoperative care after revascularization involves primarily appropriate monitoring of distal arterial flow with monitoring of pulses by palpation or Doppler ultrasound. Systemic anticoagulation is generally not indicated because of potential bleeding from local trauma and other injuries.[3,9] The orthopedic injuries generally guide rehabilitation protocols, but with appropriate care in anastomosis and grafting, the patient can be allowed to start motion fairly early. Long-term follow-up in patients with injury to one of the major arteries of the upper extremity have shown significant sequela, including reduced bone mineral density of the distal radius and decrease in grip strength.[10] Likewise those patients who suffer a concomitant nerve injury have further problems related to overall strength and function.

CLOSED INJURY

The most common closed vascular injury leading to distal ischemia is ulnar artery thrombosis or "hypothenar hammer syndrome." This occurs secondarily to trauma to the ulnar side of the palm, leading to thrombosis of the ulnar artery and distal ischemia caused by embolization of thrombus from the site of injury into (primarily) the ulnar digits of the hand. These patients are usually men who present with a history of trauma (often repeated) to the ulnar side of the palm and symptoms of ischemia of the ring and little fingers (Fig. 4).[11,12] Patients who experience repeated trauma may develop an aneurysm of the ulnar artery and develop symptoms consistent with embolization and the mass pressing on the ulnar nerve, with paresthesias and numbness in the ulnar two digits (Fig. 5).

Work-up of patients with evidence of hypothenar hammer syndrome is usually accomplished with arteriography, although computed tomography angiography and MR angiography may have some application. Arterial studies allow

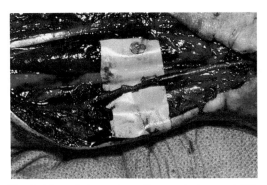

Fig. 3. View of ulnar artery after gunshot wound. This type of injury requires reversed vein grafting.

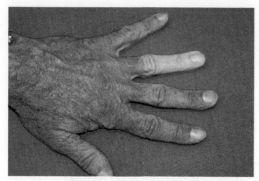

Fig. 4. Hand of 58-year-old aircraft mechanic who presented with acute onset of pain and ischemia of ring finger.

Acute ischemia from ulnar artery thrombosis can potentially be managed by thrombolysis but there are few reports of this. Up to 80% of patients in reported series do show improvement, however, and digital amputation rates are low.[13] At this time reports of successful management of thrombosis of the vessels in the hand by endovascular techniques (balloon dilitation and stents) are limited and this cannot be recommended. Many patients suffering from hypothenar hammer syndrome have severe damage to the intima, however, and I suspect that long-term patients treated without bypass have very low patency rates of the injured ulnar artery (if they do not develop an aneurysm.)

Although some patients with minimal symptoms or those that resolve may be managed nonoperatively, it is my opinion that most patients presenting with acute ischemia require exploration and excision of the damaged segment of ulnar artery with either primary repair or bypass grafting. This operation is fairly straightforward, and the ulnar artery is exposed via a Bruner incision over the course of the ulnar

delineation of the size of the occlusion and allowing for evaluation for possible aneurysm formation. Angiography typically shows an occluded ulnar artery in the palm with proximal flow via the dorsal branch proximal to the wrist or via the deep branch accompanying the motor branch of the ulnar nerve in the palm.

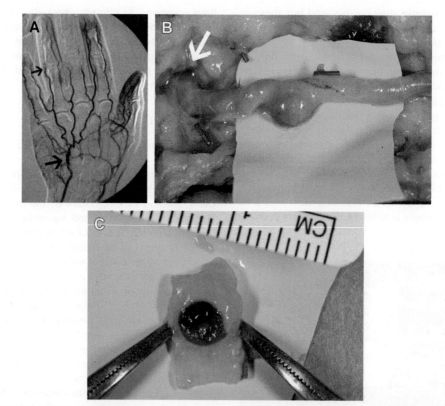

Fig. 5. (A) Arteriogram of patient presenting with symptoms of ischemia of ring and little finger. *Large arrow* shows "corkscrew" appearance of ulnar artery denoting aneurysm, *small arrow* shows blockage of digital vessel caused by embolization. (B) View of aneurysm present in this patient from chronic trauma, *arrow* points to palmar arch distal to aneurysm. (C) Aneurysm after excision showing thrombus in wall.

artery. The artery is freed up and the damaged or aneurysmal segment excised. Because of redundancy in the ulnar artery small areas of injury can occasionally be excised and primarily repaired, but most need repair with a short segment of vein graft. I prefer to use the basilic vein for this, because it is on the underside of the arm (leaving a scar that is not too visible) and is of appropriate size. Grafting proceeds as described previously.

Patients generally do well with surgical management of traumatic closed thrombosis of the ulnar artery.[11,14] Patency rates long-term are reported in the 40% to 75% range, with some evidence of a recurrence of symptoms if the bypass graft suffers thrombosis.

The radial artery in the dorsal hand can also suffer thrombosis, although this is much less common than hypothenar hammer syndrome. The cause of this seems to be compression of the radial artery by the extensor pollicis longus tendon over the trapezium. This largely occurs in women and usually causes ischemia of the index finger and thumb.[15] These patients occasionally present with a white index finger, which resolves and does not recur. I believe that this is caused by thrombosis of the radial artery with subsequent embolization to the digital vessels to the index finger without recurrence (Fig. 6). If symptoms only occur once, it is probably reasonable to place the patient on low-dose aspirin and provide close follow-up. If the finger remains ischemic it is prudent to explore the artery in the snuffbox and excise the damaged segment to prevent further embolization. Although I generally either repair this segment or vein graft it,[15] it is reasonable to simply excise the segment if there is adequate flow via the ulnar artery.[16] The graft should be placed on top

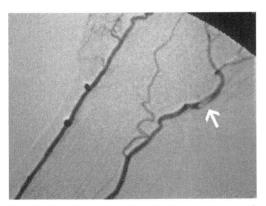

Fig. 6. Arteriography of patient presenting with ischemia of the index finger. *Arrow* points to filling defect (thrombus) in radial artery in anatomic snuffbox on dorsal wrist.

of the extensor pollicis longus (EPL) tendon or the EPL may be rerouted to prevent further compression of the graft. Recurrence rates seem to be fairly low.

OTHER CAUSES OF CLOSED ARTERIAL DAMAGE

There are several other causes of arterial damage in the upper extremity, but most of these are fairly uncommon. Fractures of various sorts can cause injury to major vessels, but unless there is a significant open injury this is unlikely to cause distal ischemia.

Fractures of the distal radius can lead to vascular injury of either the radial or ulnar arteries.[17] One study of a fairly large series of distal radius fractures by a single author found a 2% incidence of injury to the radial artery.[18] Of the two major series, however, only 50% to 70% underwent repair of the injured vessel, and patency rates were reported at 70% in one series. These injuries are probably identified more commonly now as more patients undergo open reduction and internal fixation; however, these patients rarely experience ischemia of the hand. Ligation of the injured vessel may be appropriate management in most patients.

Fractures and dislocations around the elbow are another fairly common source of arterial injuries in the upper extremity and in general the brachial artery is the vessel injured at this level. Injury to the brachial artery at the elbow level can lead to devastating consequences, including Volkmann contracture, and these injuries need to be addressed promptly.[19] Most of these injuries are caused by supracondylar fractures, but acute ischemia caused by compression of an abnormally positioned brachial artery by the lacertus fibrosis[20] and thrombosis from elbow dislocation have been reported.[21] Although the overall incidence of brachial artery injury in patients with supracondylar fracture is low, one large series of more than 1000 patients treated in a single institution found a 4% incidence of a pale, pulseless hand at presentation.[22] All of these patients had a Gartland type III fracture pattern. Only 5% of patients required vascular exploration and repair after closed reduction and percutaneous pinning. These patients had no palpable or Doppler signal in the radial pulse after reduction, and the hands remained pale. A total of 37% of the patients who initially had a pale, pulseless hand had return of capillary refill after closed reduction and percutaneous pinning (CRPP) but without palpable or Doppler pulse. All of these patients regained a palpable pulse before discharge. Color duplex scanning and ultrasound velocimetry have been shown to have some benefit in evaluating children for vascular injury and in evaluating the possible need for vascular exploration.[23,24] Other studies have confirmed that patients with a pink hand with capillary refill (and no palpable or Doppler pulses) after reduction and pinning can be safely observed[25,26]; however, some of these children develop evidence of worsening ischemia and require exploration and thus close observation is paramount. Many authors have noted the association between neurologic deficit and vascular injury in these fractures, and the absence of return of median nerve function in the forearm and hand after CRPP may be an indication for surgical exploration.[22,27] Long-term follow-up studies of patients who required revascularization has shown that growth and function are good but did note some aneurysmal change in those patients who had required vein grafting. Periodic follow-up with ultrasound to evaluate those patients with reversed vein grafts in the antecubital fossa has been proposed.[28]

Injuries to the vascular system also can occur in athletes distally and proximally. Baseball players (primarily catchers) can suffer from ischemia of the index finger of the gloved (catching) hand, and this has been noted as early as the teenage years in patients who play at a high level.[29] These patients also have an increased incidence of evidence of ulnar artery thrombosis in the catching hand. Long-term management of these patients may be difficult, because they are often professional or semiprofessional players, and stopping the offending activity may not be feasible. Better padding in the catching glove has been suggested as one way to decrease the risk of long-term sequelae.[30]

Baseball pitchers and those who perform other repetitive over-the-shoulder throwing motions are at risk of injury to the axillary artery and vein, particularly in professional or high-performance athletes (Fig. 7).[31] If this occurs with thrombosis of the axillary vein it is called Paget-Schroetter syndrome or more recently "effort thrombosis." These patients present with swelling and signs of venous occlusion of the involved extremity, and may have pain. Work-up is usually done with contrast venography but ultrasound also has been found to be useful (Fig. 8).[32] Initial management is usually performed with thrombolytics and anticoagulation. Patients with evidence of thoracic-outlet symptoms from a cervical rib usually require surgical resection of the rib, and a rare patient requires excision of the thrombosed segment of vein and vein bypass grafting. Most patients are maintained on oral anticoagulants for a period of 3 months after initial treatment, and

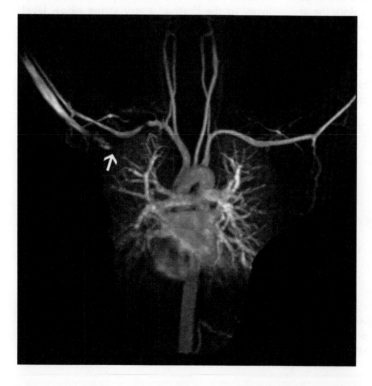

Fig. 7. MR arteriography in baseball pitcher with arms abducted. *White arrow* shows occlusion of subclavian vein and *red arrow* shows compression of subclavian artery. Patient required first rib resection. (*Courtesy of* South Texas Radiology Imaging Centers, San Antonio, TX.)

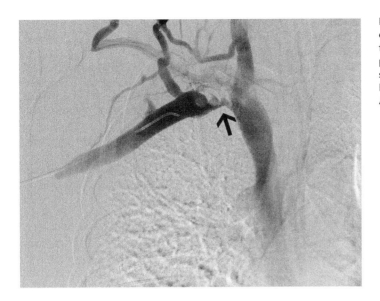

Fig. 8. Venogram of patient with effort thrombosis. *Arrow* points to thrombus in innominate vein. This patient was treated with thrombolysis. (*Courtesy of* South Texas Radiology Imaging Centers, San Antonio, TX.)

in general these patients can successfully return to high-level athletic competition.[31–33] Results of treatment seem to be predicated on the rapidity of treatment, however, with earlier management decreasing the risk of rethrombosis.[32]

Arterial injury in athletes at the level of the shoulder is often caused by thoracic outlet compression or compression of the artery by the humeral head during the throwing action.[34] These patients are usually high-level baseball pitchers and present with symptoms of arm fatigue, numbness in the hand, cold hypersensitivity, and pain.[35] These patients can develop embolization of thrombus distally, often caused by aneurysm of the circumflex humeral artery

(Fig. 9).[36] A high level of suspicion in patients who are overhead throwers who present with these symptoms is warranted, and work-up is aimed at diagnosing the site and extent of the vascular problem. This is usually done with arterial studies, and angiography is preferred because treatment can begin in the angiography suite with thrombolysis if an occlusion is identified. Management may require operative thrombectomy of distal vessels, segmental repair with reversed saphenous vein grafting, and possibly ligation and/or excision of aneurysms of the circumflex humeral artery.[35] Excision of a cervical rib causing compression of the vessel may be appropriate. Again these

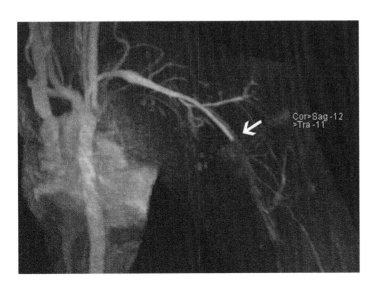

Fig. 9. MR arteriography of baseball pitcher with acute thrombosis of brachial artery. *Arrow* points to site of thrombosis, note some filling distally via collaterals. (*Courtesy of* South Texas Radiology Imaging Centers, San Antonio, TX.)

patients are generally required to avoid over-head throwing for a period of about 3 months, but somewhat surprisingly most can return to the same level of performance that they enjoyed before arterial thrombosis.

REFERENCES

1. DuBose JJ, Savage SA, Fabian TC, et al. The American Association for the Surgery of Trauma PROspective Observational Vascular Injury Treatment (PROOVIT) registry: multicenter data on modern vascular injury diagnosis, management, and outcomes. J Trauma Acute Care Surg 2015;78(2):215–22.

2. Franz RW, Skytta CK, Shah KJ, et al. A five-year review of management of upper-extremity arterial injuries at an urban level I trauma center. Ann Vasc Surg 2012;26(5):655–64.

3. Pederson WC. Replantation. Plast Reconstr Surg 2001;107(3):823–41.

4. Hornez E, Boddaert G, Baudoin Y, et al. Concomitant vascular war trauma saturating a French forward surgical team deployed to support the victims of the Syrian war (2013). Interest of the vascular damage control. Ann Vasc Surg 2015;29(8):1656.

5. Borut LT, Acosta CJ, Tadlock LC, et al. The use of temporary vascular shunts in military extremity wounds: a preliminary outcome analysis with 2-year follow-up. J Trauma 2010;69(1):174–8.

6. Gifford SM, Aidinian G, Clouse WD, et al. Effect of temporary shunting on extremity vascular injury: an outcome analysis from the Global War on Terror vascular injury initiative. J Vasc Surg 2009;50(3):549–55.

7. Nalbandian MM, Maldonado TS, Cushman J, et al. Successful limb reperfusion using prolonged intravascular shunting in a case of an unstable trauma patient–a case report. Vasc Endovascular Surg 2004;38(4):375–9.

8. Moore WS. Vascular and endovascular surgery. 8th edition. Philadelphia: Saunders Elsevier; 2013.

9. Levin LS, Cooper EO. Clinical use of anticoagulants following replantation surgery. J Hand Surg Am 2008;33(8):1437–9.

10. Sergi G, Perissinotto E, Zucchetto M, et al. Long-term outcome of morphology and function after soft tissue injury of the forearm with vascular involvement. Ann Vasc Surg 2013;27(5):599–605.

11. Kitzinger HB, van SJ, Schmitt R, et al. Hypothenar hammer syndrome: long-term results after vascular reconstruction. Ann Plast Surg 2016;76(1):40–5.

12. Scharnbacher J, Claus M, Reichert J, et al. Hypothenar hammer syndrome: a multicenter case-control study. Am J Ind Med 2013;56(11):1352–8.

13. De Martino RR, Moran SL. The role of thrombolytics in acute and chronic occlusion of the hand. Hand Clin 2015;31(1):13–21.

14. Hui-Chou HG, McClinton MA. Current options for treatment of hypothenar hammer syndrome. Hand Clin 2015;31(1):53–62.

15. McNamara MG, Butler TE, Sanders WE, et al. Ischaemia of the index finger and thumb secondary to thrombosis of the radial artery in the anatomical snuffbox. J Hand Surg Br 1998;23(1):28–32.

16. Pomahac B, Hagan R, Blazar P, et al. Spontaneous thrombosis of the radial artery at the wrist level. Plast Reconstr Surg 2004;114(4):943–6.

17. de Witte PB, Lozano-Calderon S, Harness N, et al. Acute vascular injury associated with fracture of the distal radius: a report of 6 cases. J Orthop Trauma 2008;22(9):611–4.

18. O'Toole RV, Hardcastle J, Garapati R, et al. Fracture of the distal radius with radial artery injury: injury description and outcome of vascular repair. Injury 2013;44(4):437–41.

19. Lowrie AG, Berry MG, Kirkpatrick JJ, et al. Arterial injuries at the elbow carry a high risk of muscle necrosis and warrant urgent revascularisation. Ann R Coll Surg Engl 2012;94(2):124–8.

20. De SF, Martini G, Decaminada N, et al. Arterial entrapment syndrome in the cubital fossa: a rare cause of acute stress-related arterial thrombosis in a patient with brachial artery duplication. G Chir 2012;33(11–12):383–6.

21. Garrigues GE, Patel MB, Colletti TP, et al. Thrombosis of the brachial artery after closed dislocation of the elbow. J Bone Joint Surg Br 2009;91(8):1097–9.

22. Weller A, Garg S, Larson AN, et al. Management of the pediatric pulseless supracondylar humeral fracture: is vascular exploration necessary? J Bone Joint Surg Am 2013;95(21):1906–12.

23. Benedetti VM, Martinelli O, Irace L, et al. Vascular injuries in supracondylar humeral fracture: an active approach to diagnosis and treatment. Int Angiol 2014;33(6):540–6.

24. Benedetti VM, Farsetti P, Martinelli O, et al. The value of ultrasonic diagnosis in the management of vascular complications of supracondylar fractures of the humerus in children. Bone Joint J 2013;95-B(5):694–8.

25. Wolfswinkel EM, Weathers WM, Siy RW, et al. Less is more in the nonoperative management of complete brachial artery transection after supracondylar humeral fracture. Ann Vasc Surg 2014;28(3):739–46.

26. Badkoobehi H, Choi PD, Bae DS, et al. Management of the pulseless pediatric supracondylar humeral fracture. J Bone Joint Surg Am 2015;97(11):937–43.

27. Mangat KS, Martin AG, Bache CE. The 'pulseless pink' hand after supracondylar fracture of the humerus in children: the predictive value of nerve palsy. J Bone Joint Surg Br 2009;91(11):1521–5.

28. Konstantiniuk P, Fritz G, Ott T, et al. Long-term follow-up of vascular reconstructions after supracondylar humerus fracture with vascular lesion in childhood. Eur J Vasc Endovasc Surg 2011;42(5): 684–8.

29. Sugawara M, Ogino T, Minami A, et al. Digital ischemia in baseball players. Am J Sports Med 1986;14(4):329–34.

30. Ginn TA, Smith AM, Snyder JR, et al. Vascular changes of the hand in professional baseball players with emphasis on digital ischemia in catchers. J Bone Joint Surg Am 2005;87(7):1464–9.

31. Arko FR, Harris EJ, Zarins CK, et al. Vascular complications in high-performance athletes. J Vasc Surg 2001;33(5):935–42.

32. Melby SJ, Vedantham S, Narra VR, et al. Comprehensive surgical management of the competitive athlete with effort thrombosis of the subclavian vein (Paget-Schroetter syndrome). J Vasc Surg 2008;47(4):809–20.

33. Doyle A, Wolford HY, Davies MG, et al. Management of effort thrombosis of the subclavian vein: to-day's treatment. Ann Vasc Surg 2007;21(6):723–9.

34. Rohrer MJ, Cardullo PA, Pappas AM, et al. Axillary artery compression and thrombosis in throwing athletes. J Vasc Surg 1990;11(6):761–8.

35. Duwayri YM, Emery VB, Driskill MR, et al. Positional compression of the axillary artery causing upper extremity thrombosis and embolism in the elite overhead throwing athlete. J Vasc Surg 2011;53(5): 1329–40.

36. Kee ST, Dake MD, Wolfe-Johnson B, et al. Ischemia of the throwing hand in major league baseball pitchers: embolic occlusion from aneurysms of axillary artery branches. J Vasc Interv Radiol 1995;6(6): 979–82.

Acute Carpal Tunnel Syndrome
A Review of Current Literature

Jonathan D. Gillig, MD[a], Stephen D. White, MD[a],
James Nicholas Rachel, MD[a,b,*]

KEYWORDS

- Acute carpal tunnel syndrome • Carpal tunnel syndrome • Review • Median nerve
- Wrist trauma

KEY POINTS

- Acute carpal tunnel syndrome is a known complication of wrist and hand trauma including distal radius fractures and numerous atraumatic causes.
- Patient evaluation should differentiate ACTS, which is a progressive condition from normal sensation to loss of two-point discrimination, from neuropraxic injury, which is stable loss of sensation immediately after injury.
- Complete release of the transverse carpal ligament should be performed on emergent basis after diagnosis. Concomitant fractures and underlying medical conditions should be treated as indicated.

INTRODUCTION

Carpal tunnel syndrome (CTS) is the most common peripheral nerve compression. The incidence of CTS is 99 per 100,000 individuals and it is most common in patients older than 40.[1,2] Females also comprise between 65% and 75% of all cases.[3] It is often seen as a chronic progression of median nerve compression as the nerve passes beneath the transverse carpal ligament. Although elective carpal tunnel release (CTR) is performed in severe or refractory cases, conservative management and observation are used in milder cases. Acute CTS (ACTS) is a less common presentation and requires more urgent and aggressive management. Many conditions can lead to ACTS, but central to this diagnosis is a progressive worsening of median nerve function. This is an important distinction because neuropraxia and nerve contusion can present with a similar distribution of symptoms, but their severity remains stable and does not progress over time.

The onset of ACTS is often measured in minutes to hours, in contrast to chronic CTS. ACTS most commonly results following trauma; however, numerous other etiologies have been described at a significantly lower incidence. All causes of ACTS do share the same underlying pathology of an acute increase in pressure within the carpal tunnel. This results in compromise of the epineural blood flow and thus pain and dysesthesias in the distribution of the median nerve. Urgent surgical decompression of the median nerve is necessary to prevent further progression of symptoms.

ANATOMY

The carpal tunnel is an enclosed space bordered on three sides by the carpal bones and on the fourth by the flexor retinaculum. As a result, the volume of the carpal tunnel is relatively constant at around 5 mL,[4] with little room for expansion or swelling secondary to its inelastic borders. The tunnel itself is transversed by

[a] Department of Orthopaedic Surgery, University of South Alabama School of Medicine, 3421 Medical Park Drive, Mobile, AL 36693, USA; [b] The Orthopaedic Group, P.C, 6144 Airport Boulevard, Mobile, AL 36608, USA
* Corresponding author.
E-mail address: jnickrachel@gmail.com

Orthop Clin N Am 47 (2016) 599–607
http://dx.doi.org/10.1016/j.ocl.2016.03.005
0030-5898/16/$ – see front matter © 2016 Elsevier Inc. All rights reserved.

10 structures, nine tendons and the median nerve. The tendons include the four flexor digitorum superficialis tendons, the four flexor digitorum profundus tendons, and the tendon of the flexor pollicis longus. The dorsal floor of the carpal tunnel is abutted by the triquetrum, hamate, capitate, and the scaphoid. Radially, the scaphoid tubercle and the trapezium border the tunnel with the ulnar border being composed of the triquetrum, pisiform, and the hook of the hamate. Finally, the volar surface of the tunnel is composed of three structures that make up the flexor retinaculum. These include the deep forearm fascia, the transverse carpal ligament, and the distal aponeurosis that divides the thenar and hypothenar musculature. These include the deep forearm fascia, the transverse carpal ligament, and the distal aponeurosis that divides the thenar and hypo thenar musculature (Fig. 1).

The most proximal portion of the carpal tunnel begins at the volar wrist crease and then extends distally to a line running from the abducted border of the thumb to the hook of the hamate, Kaplan cardinal line. At Kaplan cardinal line, the average width of the tunnel is 25 mm.[5] The carpal tunnel is at its narrowest, around 20 mm, at the level of the hook of the hamate. At the proximal and distal portions of the tunnel, an opening exists; however, synovium at either end results in the properties of a closed compartment. When the pressure within the compartment rises above a threshold, blood flow decreases resulting in compromise to the median nerve and paresthesias in the nerve distribution.

The median nerve supplies sensation to the most radial 3.5 fingers, the thenar musculature, and the lumbricals of the index and middle fingers. The palmar cutaneous branch of the median nerve branches off just proximal to the wrist flexion crease between the pollicis longus and the flexor carpi radialis and runs superficial to the flexor retinaculum. This nerve divides into a lateral branch, which supplies sensation over the volar base of the thumb, and the medial branch, which supplies sensation to the radial side of the palm. This sensory branch is not affected by compression in the carpal tunnel, and thus its function can help to distinguish CTS from more proximal median neuropathy. The recurrent branch of the median nerve innervates the opponens pollicis, abductor pollicis brevis, and the superficial part of the flexor pollicis brevis. The branching of this nerve has substantial anatomic variability with 50% of the population having extraligamentous branching, meaning that the motor branches occur distal to the carpal tunnel. Up to 30% of the population experiences subligamentous branching, where the motor nerve originates within the carpal tunnel. Lastly, 20% of the population experiences transligamentous branching, where the nerve branches off within the carpal tunnel and then pierces the transverse carpal ligament on its course toward the thenar musculature.[6] Other terminal branches of the median nerve include the digital cutaneous branches, which supply sensation to the radial 3.5 digits on the palmar side and the dorsal tips of the 3 most radial digits. A small percentage of 1.2% to 23% of the population may also retain the gestational remnant of the median artery, which courses with the median nerve into the hand.[7,8]

PATHOPHYSIOLOGY

Many presentations of ACTS have been reported in the literature. Although ACTS itself is uncommon, its presentation is most often considered in the setting of trauma, such as distal radius fractures or perilunate injuries. Awareness of these possible causes should guide evaluation in emergency room settings; however, small case series and case reports describe innumerable other causes ranging from gout to parvovirus. This demonstrates the importance of a thorough nerve examination in all patients with any sign of progressive nerve symptoms. The underlying pathologic process that causes ACTS is the creation of mass effect from a space-occupying lesion in the carpal tunnel resulting in increased compartmental pressures. This rise in compartmental pressure creates a compartment syndrome that results in lack of epineurial perfusion and ultimately ischemia. The lack of perfusion causes local tissue edema, nerve conduction delays propagated by demyelination along the axon, and axonal transport dysfunction that inhibits recurrent nerve firing.[9–11] Short intervals of decreased perfusion are rapidly reversible; however, a longer duration of compression increases the latency period before recovery and also increases risk of permanent disability.

Previous animal and human studies show thinned nerves in the entrapped segment with swelling of the nerve proximal to that region. This is thought to be caused by accumulation of axoplasm, nerve edema, and chronic inflammatory fibrosis of the nerve.[12,13] Demyelination and remyelination of the affected segments leads to poorer nerve conduction and a loss of large myelinated axons leading to increased latency. The normal compartment pressure of the carpal tunnel is 2.5 mm Hg at rest, and this increases with wrist flexion or extension. The average pressure is below the average capillary refill pressure of 32 mm Hg.[14] However, with forceful wrist extension and flexion, the carpal tunnel pressure can reach 30 mm Hg, and Lim and colleagues[15] showed that reduction in epineural blood flow is first noted with a carpal tunnel pressure of 20 to 30 mm Hg. Thus, a compartment pressure of 30 mm Hg can lead to the development of neuronal changes. It has also been shown that the microscopic changes occur in a dose-dependent manner with increased time periods of high pressure resulting in increased latency and more permanent damage.[16]

Extension and flexion of the wrist also causes a decrease in the cross-sectional area of the carpal tunnel. With wrist extension, the narrowing occurs at the level of the pisiform. Wrist flexion results in narrowing at the level of the hook of the hamate.[17] Wrist flexion also results in the retraction of the transverse carpal ligament to a position that is closer to the distal radius, which results in a further decrease in area.

ETIOLOGY

Acute carpal tunnel syndrome most often occurs following traumatic injury to the patient's wrist or hand, however numerous atraumatic causes have been described in the literature and providers must keep these alternatives in mind. A schematic diagram of the variable etiologies will be discussed further in the following sections and can be easily visualized in Fig. 2.

Traumatic

Following any significant wrist or hand trauma, ACTS must be ruled out, because it is a common complication. High-energy injuries in young patients have the highest risk of developing ACTS. In fact, ACTS was first described by Paget in 1853 in a patient who had suffered a distal radius fracture and suffered rapidly progressive neuropathy. It is important to differentiate nerve contusion from ACTS initially, because the management differs significantly. Often a complete history and serial examinations can help to distinguish the two. Mack and colleagues report key differences between these two conditions. Patients with ACTS have a normal median nerve examination initially with progression to loss of two-point discrimination. In contrast, patients with nerve contusions experience immediate, but nonprogressive and static sensory loss. In ACTS, intercarpal pressure measurements were also shown to be elevated in contrast to normal levels in nerve contusion.

Distal radius fractures are one of the more common associated injuries with ACTS (Figs. 2 and 3). A study by Dyer and colleagues[18] looked at predictors of ACTS associated with distal radius fractures. Out of 50 patients who had concurrent ACTS and distal radius fractures, translation of fracture greater than 35% and female age less than 48 years were the most highly correlated risk factors for ACTS development. Dyer put the incidence of ACTS in the setting of distal radius fractures at 5.4%, whereas several older

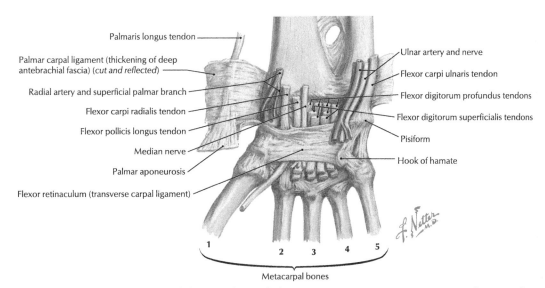

Palmaris longus tendon

Palmar carpal ligament (thickening of deep antebrachial fascia) (cut and reflected)

Radial artery and superficial palmar branch

Flexor carpi radialis tendon

Flexor pollicis longus tendon

Median nerve

Palmar aponeurosis

Flexor retinaculum (transverse carpal ligament)

Ulnar artery and nerve

Flexor carpi ulnaris tendon

Flexor digitorum profundus tendons

Flexor digitorum superficialis tendons

Pisiform

Hook of hamate

1 2 3 4 5

Metacarpal bones

Fig. 1. Volar anatomic diagram of the carpal tunnel demonstrating compartment contents and surrounding structures.

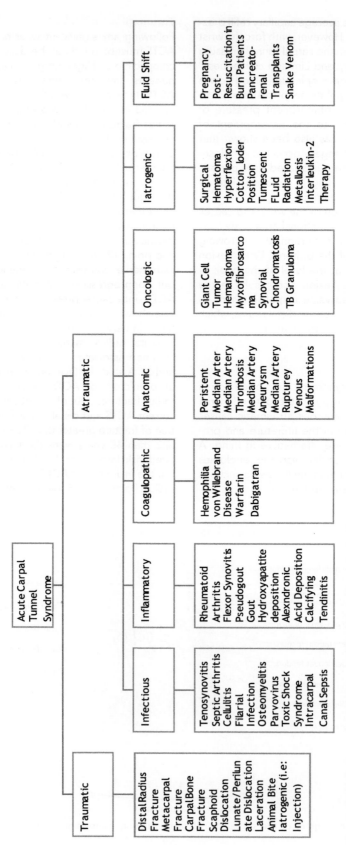

Fig. 2. Described causes of acute carpal tunnel syndrome in the literature.

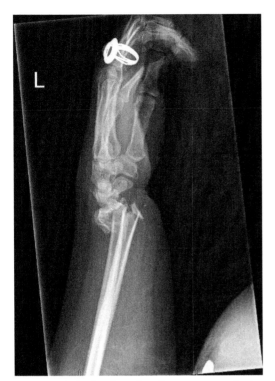

Fig. 3. ACTS distal radius fracture prereduction lateral.

studies cited the incidence as between 0.2% and 21.5%.[19] The cause of these traumatic ACTS is most likely secondary to hemorrhage into the tunnel at the fracture site. The former practice of splinting wrists in the Cotton-Loder position, which involved significant wrist flexion, has also been implicated in increasing the incidence of ACTS following distal radius fractures.[20]

Other trauma to the hand including carpal fractures, dislocations, fracture-dislocations, and iatrogenic causes has been associated with ACTS. Volar fracture and subluxation of the bases of the second and third metacarpals into the carpal tunnel have been reported as causes of ACTS.[21] Other case reports describe ACTS following nondisplaced fractures of the scaphoid and fifth metacarpal.[22] This demonstrates the mass effect component secondary to swelling that can cause ACTS and not just fracture fragments infringing on the tunnel. Another case report in 2010 describes how traumatic iatrogenic causes can result in ACTS. In this case, a patient on anticoagulation with an unsuccessful arterial line placement developed ACTS and forearm compartment syndrome. In this case, 20 mL of blood and blood clots were removed from the carpal tunnel on urgent exploration. This patient's symptoms progressed over approximately 12 hours and resulted in residual median neuropathy but improved hand function.[23]

Atraumatic

The atraumatic causes of ACTS are almost innumerable. Many case reports have been written regarding a variety of causes of atraumatic ACTS and new causes will likely arise in the future. Fortunately, atraumatic ACTS is a rare entity. The goal in this article is not to mention every cause of ACTS, but rather to build a framework that helps to classify the varying causes into categories to help diagnosticians when encountering a patient with symptoms consistent with ACTS.

Infectious causes of ACTS are varied and include viral, bacterial, and parasitic origins. In all instances, the body's inflammatory response to these foreign organisms can create increased pressure within the carpal tunnel leading to sudden onset of symptoms. With nine tendons traversing the carpal tunnel, infectious tenosynovitis of the flexor tendons is one atraumatic cause that can affect any of the tendon sheaths. Case reports identifying the causative organism have included *Staphylococcus aureus*, mycobacterium, *Histoplasma capsulatum*, cryptococcus, *Neisseria gonorrhea*, and *Brucella*.[24] Case reports involving septic arthritis,[25] parvovirus infection,[26] filarial infection,[27] and even a case of a cat bite[28] have all demonstrated different infectious processes that can lead to ACTS.

Noninfectious inflammatory causes of ACTS is another category to be discussed. These conditions range from flexor synovitis,[29] to gout[30] and pseudogout,[31] to rheumatoid arthritis.[32]

Coagulopathies, whether congenital or medication induced, have been implicated in ACTS. In these patients, even trivial injury can result in hematoma formation.[33] With an aging population and increasing numbers of people requiring anticoagulation, this is a cause that needs to be considered more frequently. Even newer generations of anticoagulants, such as dabigatran, increase the risk of bleeding and can thus result in ACTS.[34]

Individuals with anatomic anomalies and pathology have also been implicated in ACTS. Patients with a persistent median artery have been reported to develop ACTS following median artery thrombosis, aneurysm, and rupture.[35–38] Venous malformations in patients have also been reported causes.[39]

Iatrogenic causes of ACTS can be traumatic and atraumatic. Postsurgical hematoma is a common cause that must be looked for in the postoperative period. One case report of ACTS occurred in a total wrist arthroplasty patient 6 years postoperatively from metallosis of the components.[40] A far less common cause includes tumescence fluid being injected into the carpal tunnel during burn surgery.[41] Lastly, a case of ACTS was reported in a patient who was undergoing radiation therapy for a high-grade sarcoma on his right hand.[42]

Large shifts in body fluids have also resulted in ACTS, such as during pregnancy[43] and in postresuscitative burn patients.[44] Other rare case reports, such as in pancreatic-renal transplants[45] and in patients exposed to snake venom,[46] result from third spacing of fluids.

Lastly, oncologic causes of ACTS are another category to be aware of. These are more likely to be of gradual onset and thus more likely fall into the category of CTS but they are included here for completeness. A study by Martínez-Villén and colleagues[47] demonstrated these symptoms in patients with diagnoses including a giant cell tumor of a tendon sheath, synovial chondromatosis, tuberculosis granuloma, and tophaceous gout.

DIAGNOSIS

Physical Examination

A thorough physical examination with monitoring over time remains the best avenue for diagnosing ACTS. The evaluating physician must be diligent in the evaluation of the patient's neurovascular status and maintain a high level of clinical suspicion for ACTS similar to compartment syndrome in injuries that predispose patients to this condition. Nerve contusion must be distinguished from progressive neuropraxia in the median nerve distribution. Nerve contusion is represented by static symptoms that gradually improve over time. ACTS instead presents as initially paresthesias and dysesthesias that progress with increasingly worsening two-point discrimination. As untreated ACTS progresses, the patient loses all sensation distal to the carpal tunnel in the median nerve distribution and often experiences loss of grip strength. Physical examination maneuvers, such as Phalen, Tinel, and Durkan, can further exacerbate ACTS progression, and thus their use should be limited. Lastly, compartment pressure monitoring provides the most objective measure to determine increased carpal tunnel pressures. Pressures greater than 20 mm Hg have demonstrated decreased epineuronal blood flow with pressures closer to 30 mm Hg resulting in neuronal

changes. The widespread adoption of these monitoring devices has been limited by the sensitivity of a good physical examination in diagnosing ACTS.

Imaging

ACTS does not in itself require specific imaging because it is based on a clinical evaluation. Radiographs should be standard in the management of cases secondary to trauma. Dyer demonstrated that distal radius fracture translation was the most important factor leading to ACTS (**Figs. 3** and **4**). The increased risk in women younger than 48 and those with greater than 35% fracture translation can be helpful when evaluating patients. Prophylactic CTR may be appropriate in this group; however, ACTS remains a clinical diagnosis that must be monitored over time. Advanced imaging, such as MRI or computed tomography, can be used if needed in a case of trauma for preoperative planning. They may also be required for more atypical causes, such as masses or infections. These advanced imaging techniques have been helpful from a research standpoint in determining carpal tunnel physiology and mechanics during wrist motion. Nonetheless, it is important to remember that emergent CTR should not be significantly delayed for these tests because it could lead to irreversible median nerve damage.

Treatment

Complete release of the transverse carpal ligament is usually the required treatment of

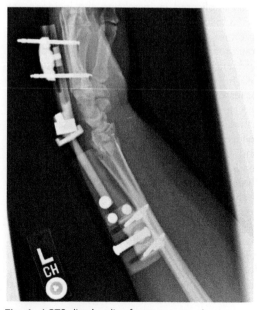

Fig. 4. ACTS distal radius fracture postreduction.

ACTS. This procedure is performed through an open technique via a palmar incision. Similar to an elective CTR, the incision should be made in line with the radial border of the ring finger or ulnar border of the palmaris longus to prevent injury to the palmar cutaneous branch and recurrent motor branch of the median nerve. Often this is performed through a more extensile incision than for an elective CTR. This allows for better visualization because of significant swelling that is often present after acute injury. It also allows the surgeon to address other underlying pathology, such as a mass or fracture/dislocation. The incision may be carried 2 cm proximal to wrist flexion crease for perilunate dislocation[48] or further proximal as necessary for treatment of a distal radius fracture.[49] It is important that a complete release of the transverse carpal ligament be performed, which is another reason visualization needs to be optimal. Care should be taken at the distal aspect of the incision as not to cause injury to the transverse arch. Special attention should also be directly ulnarly so as not to risk injury to the ulnar neurovascular bundle. One must also be cognizant of retractor placement, particularly with retracting along the radial aspect of the median nerve because this can result in injury to the recurrent motor branch.[48]

Surgical timing is as important as complete release of the carpal ligament. Outcomes of many case series show delayed release leads to irreversible damage and intraneural fibrosis.[50,51] These reports have not recommended a specific time frame for release. However, ACTS should be viewed as a surgical urgency if not an emergency, with release when an operating room is available and the patient is stable for surgery. In the setting of wrist or hand trauma, a closed reduction should first be attempted of any displaced fractures or dislocations. The wrist should then be placed in a neutral position followed by strict elevation. Mack and colleagues suggested if pain and progressive median nerve dysfunction persist for 2 hours after presentation and reduction, then intracarpal pressure should be checked. In pressure readings 40 mm Hg and greater, a CTR is performed emergently within 8 hours of onset. If pressures are normal, continued observation is recommended.

Although ACTS typically results from trauma, it can possibly result from an underlying medical cause. In these instances, the treatment typically requires more than a simple CTR but also appropriate medical treatments for such conditions as gout or bleeding disorders. There have been several case reports of ACTS caused by anticoagulants; many of these show varying treatment approaches.[34,52–56] For instance, Black and colleagues[52] suggest maintaining international normalized ratio and not stopping therapy, whereas Bonatz and colleagues[54] suggest reversing the anticoagulant if possible and attempting conservative treatment. One must be cautious when attempting conservative management, however, because of the possible perilous consequences of delayed treatment, such as prolonged or incomplete recovery and possible increased risk of early reflex sympathetic dystrophy.[34,54,55] Early surgical intervention has been shown to have rapid and full recovery of median nerve function.[34,52,55] Sibley and Mandel[34] in a case report showed a patient who developed ACTS after dabigatran therapy and underwent emergent CTR with complete recovery of median nerve. They recommended prompt surgical decompression in cases of ACTS caused by bleeding. In these less common situations where there is a medical cause, it is important to take a multidisciplinary approach to fully treat the patient's condition. After the appropriate urgent surgical management has been undertaken, this may require consulting physicians with the proper expertise to make sure the patient's medical management is optimized.

Outcomes

On review of published literature, outcomes are related to timely CTR. If CTR is performed early, the nerve often recovers fully. If delayed, irreversible nerve damage can lead to permanent nerve impairment. However, there is no consensus presented in the literature on a recommended time window from onset to release. Bauman and colleagues[50] and Ford and Ali[51] demonstrated in case series that delayed intervention of only 36 to 96 hours can have permanent consequences. Mack and colleagues recommended release within 8 hours of onset to improve outcomes. Outcomes vary in atraumatic and medical cases based to some degree on the time from onset to treatment and the underlying pathology that precipitated the ACTS. Larger series are reported in cases secondary to trauma. Chauhan and colleagues[57] retrospectively compared outcomes of acute CTR in combination with open reduction internal fixation of distal radius fractures and elective CTR. They found no long-term differences in Boston Carpal Tunnel Questionnaire scores, symptom severity, and functional status. Obviously other than timely treatment, there is certainly an element of the severity of the underlying cause that affects outcomes, although this has not been specifically addressed in the literature. This particularly applies to traumatic causes, with higher energy injuries with more displacement likely being related to worse outcomes.

SUMMARY

ACTS is a progressive median nerve compression leading to loss of two-point discrimination. Most cases encountered are in the emergency department following wrist trauma and distal radius fractures. Although rare, atraumatic and medical cases have been reported and diligent evaluation of these patients should be performed. If missed or neglected irreversible damage could occur to the median nerve. Once diagnosed, emergent CTR should be performed. If performed in a timely manner outcomes are excellent, often with complete recovery.

REFERENCES

1. Szabo RM, Madison M. Carpal tunnel syndrome. Orthop Clin North Am 1992;23:103–9.

2. von Schroeder HP, Botte MJ. Carpal tunnel syndrome. Hand Clin 1996;12:643–55.

3. Phalen GS. The carpal-tunnel syndrome. J Bone Joint Surg Am 1966;48-A:211–28.

4. Rotman MB, Donovan JP. Practical anatomy of the carpal tunnel. Hand Clin 2002;18:219–30.

5. Cobb T, Dalley B, Posteraro R, et al. Anatomy of the flexor retinaculum. J Hand Surg 1993;18:91–9.

6. Mitchell R, Chesney A, Seal S, et al. Anatomical variations of the carpal tunnel structures. Can J Plast Surg 2009;17(3):e3–7.

7. Bilgin SS, Olcay SE, Derincek A, et al. Can simple release relieve symptoms of carpal tunnel syndrome caused by a persistent median artery? Arch Orthop Trauma Surg 2004;124:154–6.

8. Olave E, Prates JC, Gabrielli C, et al. Median artery and superficial palmar branch of the radial artery in the carpal tunnel. Scand J Plast Reconstr Surg Hand Surg 1997;31:13–6.

9. Fowler TJ, Ochoa J. Recovery of nerve conduction after pneumatic tourniquet: observations on the hindlimb of the baboon. J Neurol Neurosurg Psychiatry 1975;35:638–45.

10. Ochoa J, Fowler TJ, Gilliat RW. Anatomical changes in peripheral nerve lesions compressed by a pneumatic tourniquet. J Anat 1972;113:433–55.

11. Rudge P, Ochoa J, Gilliatt RW. Acute peripheral nerve compression in the baboon. J Neurol Sci 1974;23:403.

12. Thomas PK, Fullerton PM. Nerve fiber size in the carpal tunnel syndrome. J Neurol Neurosurg Psychiatry 1963;26:520.

13. Rydevik B, McLean WG, Sjö strand J, et al. Blockage of axonal transport induced by acute, graded compression of the rabbit vagus nerve. J Neurol Neurosurg Psychiatry 1980;43:690–8.

14. Gelberman RH, Hergenroeder PT, Hargens AR, et al. The carpal tunnel syndrome: a study of carpal tunnel pressures. J Bone Joint Surg Am 1981;63: 380–3.

15. Lim JY, Cho S-H, Han TR, et al. Dose-responsiveness of electrophysiologic change in a new model of acute carpal tunnel syndrome. Clin Orthop Relat Res 2004;427:120–6.

16. Lundborg G. Ischemic nerve injury. Experimental studies on intraneural microvascular pathophysiology and nerve function in a limb subjected to temporary circulatory arrest. Scand J Plast Reconstr Surg Suppl 1970;6:3–113.

17. Yoshioka S, Okuda Y, Tamai K, et al. Changes in carpal tunnel shape during wrist joint motions. J Hand Surg 1994;18B:620–3.

18. Dyer G, Lozano-Calderon S, Gannon C, et al. Predictors of acute carpal tunnel syndrome associated with fracture of the distal radius. J Hand Surg 2008; 33(8):1309–13.

19. Mack GR, McPherson SA, Lutz RB. Acute median neuropathy after wrist trauma: the role of emergent carpal tunnel release. Clin Orthop Relat Res 1994; 300:141–6, 1124.

20. Abbott LC, Saunders JB. Injuries of the median nerve in fractures of the lower end of the radius. Surg Gynecol Obstet 1933;57:507–16.

21. Weiland AJ, Lister GD, Villarreal-Rios A. Volar fracture dislocations of the second and third carpometacarpal joints associated with acute carpal tunnel syndrome. J Trauma 1976;16:672–5.

22. Olerud C, Lonnquist L. Acute carpal tunnel syndrome caused by fracture of the scaphoid and the 5th metacarpal bones. Injury 1984;16:198–9.

23. Kokosis G, Blueschke G, Blanton M, et al. Acute carpal tunnel syndrome secondary to iatrogenic hemorrhage. A case report. Hand 2010;6(2):206–8.

24. Nourissat G, Fournier E, Werther JR, et al. Acute carpal tunnel syndrome secondary to pyogenic tenosynovitis. J Hand Surg Br 2006;31(6):687–8.

25. Gerardi JA, Mack GR, Lutz RB. Acute carpal tunnel syndrome secondary to septic arthritis of the wrist. J Am Osteopath Assoc 1989;89(7):933–4.

26. Samii K, Cassinotti P, de Freudenreich J, et al. Acute bilateral carpal tunnel syndrome associated with human parvovirus B19 infection. Clin Infect Dis 1996;22(1):162–4.

27. Gallagher B, Khalifa M, Van Heerden P, et al. Acute carpal tunnel syndrome due to filarial infection. Pathol Res Pract 2002;198(1):65–7.

28. Sbai MA, Dabloun S, Benzarti S, et al. Acute carpal tunnel syndrome of the hand following a cat bite. Pan Afr Med J 2015;21:206.

29. Shimizu A, Ikeda M, Kobayashi Y, et al. Carpal tunnel syndrome with wrist trigger caused by

hypertrophied lumbrical muscle and tenosynovitis. Case Rep Orthop 2015;2015:705237, 3 pages.

30. Pai CH, Tseng CH. Acute carpal tunnel syndrome caused by tophaceous gout. J Hand Surg Am 1993;18(4):667–9.

31. Chiu KY, Ng WF, Wong WB, et al. Acute carpal tunnel syndrome caused by pseudogout. J Hand Surg Am 1992;17(2):299–302.

32. McClain EJ, Wissinger HA. The acute carpal tunnel syndrome: nine case reports. J Trauma 1976;16(1):75–8.

33. Mayne AI, Howard A, Kent M, et al. Acute carpal tunnel syndrome in a patient with haemophilia. Case Rep 2012;2012 [pii:bcr0320126152].

34. Sibley PA, Mandel RJ. Atraumatic acute carpal tunnel syndrome in a patient taking dabigatran. Orthopedics 2012;35(8):e1286–9.

35. Dickinson JC, Kleinert JM. Acute carpal tunnel syndrome caused by a calcified median artery: a case report. J Bone Joint Surg Am 1991;73:610–1.

36. Faithfull DK, Wallace RF. Traumatic rupture of median artery: an unusual cause for acute median nerve compression. J Hand Surg Br 1987; 12:233–5.

37. Rose RE. Acute carpal tunnel syndrome secondary to thrombosis of a persistent median artery. West Indian Med J 1995;44:32–3.

38. Wright C, MacFarlane I. Aneurysm of the median artery causing carpal tunnel syndrome. Aust N Z J Surg 1994;64:66–7.

39. Hariri A, Cohen G, Masmejean EH. Venous malformation involving median nerve causing acute carpal tunnel syndrome. J Hand Surg Eur Vol 2011;36(5):431–2.

40. Day CS, Lee AH, Ahmed I. Acute carpal tunnel secondary to metallosis after total wrist arthroplasty. J Hand Surg Eur Vol 2013;38(1):80–1.

41. Al-Hassani F, Amin K, Lo S. Burns from acetylene gas: more than skin deep. BMJ Case Rep 2014; 2014 [pii:bcr2013200007].

42. Franco J, Kumpf AS, Ferguson JS. Acute carpal tunnel syndrome secondary to radiation treatment: a case report. Can J Plast Surg 2009;17(4):e35–6.

43. Bhardwaj A, Nagandla K. Musculoskeletal symptoms and orthopaedic complications in pregnancy: pathophysiology, diagnostic approaches and modern management. Postgrad Med J 2014;90(1066):450–60.

44. Balakrishnan C, Mussman JL, Balakrishnan A, et al. Acute carpal tunnel syndrome from burns of the hand and wrist. Can J Plast Surg 2009; 17(4):e33–4.

45. Mahmud T. Bilateral acute carpal tunnel syndrome after combined pancreatic and renal transplant. Scand J Plast Reconstr Surg Hand Surg 2009; 43(3):174–6.

46. Schweitzer G, Lewis JS. Puff adder bite–an unusual cause of bilateral carpal tunnel syndrome. A case report. S Afr Med J 1981;60(18):714–5.

47. Martínez-Villén G, Badiola J, Alvarez-Alegret R, et al. Nerve compression syndromes of the hand and forearm associated with tumours of non-neural origin and tumour-like lesions. J Plast Reconstr Aesthet Surg 2014;67(6):828–36.

48. Stannard JP, Schmidt AH, Kregor PJ. Surgical treatment of orthopaedic trauma. New York: Thieme; 2007. p. 400.

49. Lewis MH. Median nerve decompression after Colles's fracture. J Bone Joint Surg Br 1978;60-B(2):195–6.

50. Bauman TD, Gelberman RH, Mubarak SJ, et al. The acute carpal tunnel syndrome. Clin Orthop 1981; 156:151–6.

51. Ford DJ, Ali MS. Acute carpal tunnel syndrome: complications of delayed decompression. J Bone Joint Surg Br 1986;68-B(5):758–9.

52. Black PR, Flowers MJ, Saleh M. Acute carpal tunnel syndrome as a complication of oral anticoagulant therapy. J Hand Surg Br 1997;22:50–1.

53. Bindiger A, Zelnik J, Kuschner S; et al. Spontaneous acute carpal tunnel syndrome in an anticoagulated patient. Bull Hosp Jt Dis 1995;54:52–3.

54. Bonatz E, Seabol KE. Acute carpal tunnel syndrome in a patient taking Coumadin: case report. J Trauma 1993;35:143–4, 7.

55. Copeland J, Wells HG Jr, Puckett CL. Acute carpal tunnel syndrome in a patient taking Coumadin. J Trauma 1989;29:131–2.

56. Dussa CU, Gul A. An unusual cause of acute carpal tunnel syndrome. Acta Orthop Belg 2005; 71:236–8.

57. Chauhan A, Bowlin TC, Mih AD, et al. Patient-reported outcomes after acute carpal tunnel release in patients with distal radius open reduction internal fixation. Hand 2012;7(2):147–50.

Compartment Syndrome of the Hand

Nikhil R. Oak, MD[a], Reid A. Abrams, MD[b],*

KEYWORDS

• Compartment syndrome • Hand • Upper extremity • Hand surgery

KEY POINTS

- Many etiologies can create increased compartmental pressure, which causes capillary bed collapse, decreased tissue perfusion, and cell death.
- Examination findings of disproportionate pain, hand swelling, intrinsic minus posturing, and intracompartmental pressure monitoring aid in the diagnosis.
- Early recognition and compartment release can minimize functional loss.
- Emergency fasciotomy is the definitive treatment for hand compartment syndrome.

INTRODUCTION

Hand compartment syndrome is a relatively uncommon condition, with many etiologies, and if not diagnosed and managed expeditiously, results in significant functional morbidity. Early recognition is crucial to initiating timely treatment and minimizing functional loss. There are numerous etiologies of compartment syndrome including trauma, insect bites, high-pressure injection, infection, contrast infusion, and crush injuries[1–12] (Box 1).

Pathophysiology

Although underlying causes vary, the final common pathophysiologic pathway of compartment syndrome is increased compartmental content resulting in increased interstitial fluid pressure, which causes capillary bed collapse, decreased tissue perfusion, and cell death.[13] A vicious cycle occurs where increased intracompartmental pressure leads to decreased tissue perfusion, increased capillary permeability, and, in turn, interstitial fluid leaks into the compartment, amplifying intracompartmental pressure, and so on. The magnitude and duration of the compartmental pressure influences tissue viability (Fig. 1).

Nerve axonal transport slows with a pressure of 30 mm Hg.[14] Nerve conduction disturbance can occur with pressures within 30 mm Hg below the diastolic blood pressure, with conduction stopping at 50 mm Hg.[15–18] Gelberman and colleagues[17] discussed both motor and sensory responses of nerves were completely blocked at a threshold of 50 mm Hg. The critical pressure threshold found in the canine model for ischemic muscle necrosis was 20 mm Hg less than the diastolic blood pressure.[19] In human subjects, the progression of neuromuscular deterioration (with compartment pressure of 35–40 mm Hg less than diastolic blood pressure) was, in order: gradual loss of sensation, subjective complaints of pain, reduced nerve conduction velocity, decreased muscle action potential amplitude, and motor weakness.[18]

Reversible muscle damage occurs after 4 hours of compression and it becomes irreversible by 8 hours.[20]

The normal compartment pressures can vary between individuals with normal interstitial fluid pressures between 0 and 25.2 mm Hg.[21–23] In canine studies,[15,24] ischemia and abnormal metabolism occurs with pressures within 20[15] to 30[24] mm Hg of diastolic blood pressure. When tissue pressures reach this threshold,

---

[a] Department of Orthopaedic Surgery, University of California, San Diego, 200 West Arbor Drive, #8670, San Diego, CA 92103-8670, USA; [b] Hand, Upper Extremity, and Microvascular Surgery, Department of Orthopaedic Surgery, University of California, San Diego, 200 West Arbor Drive, #8670, San Diego, CA 92103-8670, USA
* Corresponding author.
E-mail address: raabrams@ucsd.edu

Orthop Clin N Am 47 (2016) 609–616
http://dx.doi.org/10.1016/j.ocl.2016.03.006
0030-5898/16/$ – see front matter © 2016 Elsevier Inc. All rights reserved.

extraluminal pressure will cause vascular collapse and tissue hypoxia.[13,25] Whitesides and associates[26] discussed the experimental and clinical techniques of measuring tissue pressures within a closed compartment, and noted that inadequate perfusion and relative ischemia was found if the compartment pressure was within 30 mm Hg of the patient's diastolic blood pressure. Most authors agree and recommend releasing compartments when compartment pressures are within 30 mm Hg of the diastolic pressure when subjective and physical examination signs are unreliable.[15,26–29]

Anatomy

Compartments are defined as enclosed myofascial spaces bound by thicker connective tissues or bones.[5,13,25] The myofascial spaces in the hand are the hypothenar, thenar, adductor, carpal canal, finger, and 4 interosseous compartments.[30,31] The hand itself in cross-section can be divided into 10 compartments (Fig. 2).

The thenar compartment consists of the abductor pollicis brevis, opponens pollicis, and flexor pollicis brevis innervated by the recurrent median nerve with some contributions from the ulnar nerve. The abductor digiti minimi, flexor digiti minimi, and opponens digiti minimi comprise the hypothenar muscles, innervated by the ulnar nerve. The adductor compartment consists of the adductor pollicis between the volar interossei and the lumbricals on the radial side of the hand. There are 4 dorsal and 3 volar interosseous muscles that have been identified as each distinct compartments that can show variations[31] whose physiologic relevance must be confirmed clinically.[5,32] Ling and Kumar[33] postulate that the overlying skin can serve as a constrictive layer in addition to thicker fascial compartments that contributes to increased intracompartmental pressures. The carpal canal, although not a separate muscular compartment, is a defined space that with swelling or fracture can present with median nerve compression and acute carpal tunnel

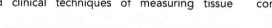

Compartment Syndrome Pathophysiology

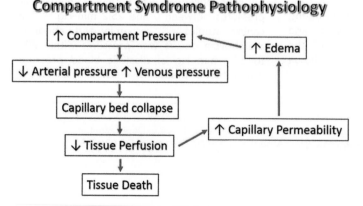

Fig. 1. Compartment syndrome pathophysiology. ↓, decreased; ↑, increased.

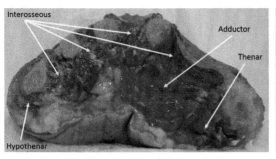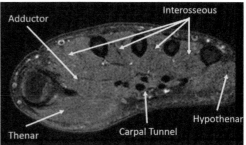

Fig. 2. Cross-sectional anatomy of the hand. Anatomic specimen on the left and cross-sectional T2 weighted MRI image on the right.

syndrome.[12] The fingers can also develop compartment syndrome with excessive swelling, often associated with burns, within the fascial compartments bound by skin and Cleland's and Grayson's ligaments.[34]

PATIENT EVALUATION

Early recognition is vital to minimize tissue necrosis and functional loss. In a cooperative patient, compartment syndrome can usually be diagnosed by history and physical examination. Taking a history including injury mechanism is important. Compartment syndrome is associated with high-energy trauma, such as motor vehicle collision, fall from height, or crush injuries. Prolonged compression under a heavy object or the patient's body, as can occur with drug overdose or positioning during a prolonged surgery are also risk factors.[35]

Historically, the 5 *Ps*—pain, pallor, paresthesias, paralysis, and pulselessness[36]—have been considered the diagnostic physical findings of compartment syndrome. Disproportionate pain is the most reliable.[20,30,34] In actuality, the remaining *Ps* are confounding because they are not always present, and their absence does not rule compartment syndrome out. The 5 *Ps* are more useful features of a vascular injury, rather than compartment syndrome. Pallor and pulselessness are present after a vascular injury, and can occur in the absence of compartment syndrome. Alternatively, there can be increased pressure in an underlying compartment despite good skin color, owing to perfusion of the skin via the dermal plexus. The presence of a pulse does not rule out compartment syndrome because the critical compartment pressure is capillary filling pressure, which is lower than arterial pressure. Compartment syndrome is often present despite the presence of a pulse. Parasthesias may occur coincidentally with compartment syndrome, but may not; it depends on whether a sensory nerve

traverses the involved compartment. The absence of parasthesia does not rule out a compartment syndrome. The paralysis associated with compartment syndrome is more likely pseudoparalysis owing to poor recruitment from severe pain rather than motor nerve compression, at least in earlier stages. Later in the disease process, paralysis can evolve from nerve and muscle ischemia. Untreated and late in the process, after muscle death, fibrotic muscle becomes contracted resulting in intrinsic plus posturing.

Acute hand compartment syndrome presents with intrinsic minus posturing, and substantial swelling (**Fig. 3**). Interphalangeal motion and adduction/abduction of digits is painful.

If present, digital parasthesias result from nerve compression or ischemia. Sometimes sensory disturbances are the first clinical symptoms mediated by dysfunction of unmyelinated sensory fibers most sensitive to hypoxia.[20] Examination of light touch, 2-point discrimination, and motor function can help to measure these early disturbances. Palpable swelling, firmness, and skin tension, with loss of normal skin creases and pallor as a result of edema and skin hypoperfusion, can all be present.

A high index of suspicion is necessary in settings where taking a history or physical examination may not be possible. Intracompartmental pressure monitoring is necessary in these situations, such as in the unconscious patient or the patient with a head injury, acute intoxication, regional anesthesia, nerve injury, or in children. Many measurement techniques have been described. Whitesides and colleagues[26] first pioneered indirect interstitial monitoring and Matsen and colleagues[37] introduced continuous indirect monitoring. Indirect monitoring refers to the compartment pressure calculated by measuring the pressure needing to overcome direct injection of a small amount of fluid into the compartment. The wick catheter, described by Mubarak and colleagues,[38] has small

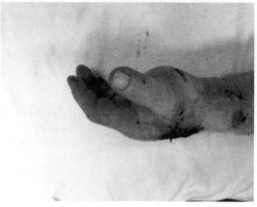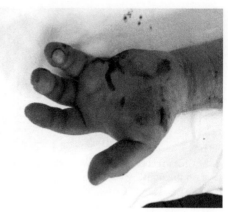

Fig. 3. Acute hand compartment syndrome in a patient which exhibits common posturing and substantial swelling. Of note, patient has had a previous ray resection.

filaments on the tip to prevent occlusion of the catheter tip by soft tissue that would prevent pressure measurement, and was initially developed for measurement of subcutaneous pressure and later adapted to directly measure and continuously monitor intramuscular pressure. A catheter modification was subsequently described, the slit catheter, which functions similarly to the wick catheter and also allows direct pressure monitoring.[39] Handheld, battery-operated devices allowing for direct compartment pressure measurement are commonly used today (Fig. 4).

The compartment being measured should be at the level of the heart and evaluated individually, with the needle inserted perpendicular to the skin.[28] "Control" pressure measurements can be made in the soft tissue outside of each compartment (Fig. 5).

The needle can then be inserted into the compartment, in the dorsal hand 1 cm proximal to the metacarpal head in the muscle belly for dorsal interosseous compartments. When the same needle is advanced 1 cm deeper, the volar interosseous compartment can be measured. The needle can be placed in the substance of the thumb–index webspace for the adductor compartment measurement. For thenar and

hypothenar measurements, the needle is placed over the maximum bulk of muscle at the glaborous skin junction.[28]

Ouellette and Kelly[8] used subjective findings, intrinsic minus posturing and suggested a threshold pressure of 15 to 25 mm Hg as diagnostic. Wong and colleagues[40] noted that subjective examination assessment of compartment tightness was insufficient to detect increased compartment pressures in the hands, advocating that handheld manometry significantly increased sensitivity and accuracy in diagnosing compartment syndrome. Based on a current understanding of tissue metabolism and muscle ischemia, especially with an unreliable examination or unclear clinical scenario, it has been recommended that hand compartments should be released when pressures are within 30 mm Hg of the patient's diastolic blood pressure or higher.[27] When pressure in a single compartment is elevated, all compartments, including the carpal tunnel, should be released.[28]

If compartment syndrome is not diagnosed clinically or by pressure measurements, but remains a worry based on mechanism or initial presentation, the patient should continue to be closely observed with serial examinations. The arm should be elevated and any constrictive bandages and intravenous access lines should be removed from the affected extremity. Fluid balance needs to be closely monitored medically. There has been scarce evidence for diuresis for treatment of impending compartment syndrome.[41]

TREATMENT

Emergency fasciotomy is the definitive treatment for hand compartment syndrome. Through longitudinal skin incisions, the fascia is widely

Fig. 4. Stryker intracompartmental pressure monitor. (*Courtesy of* Stryker Corporation, Kalamazoo, MI; with permission.)

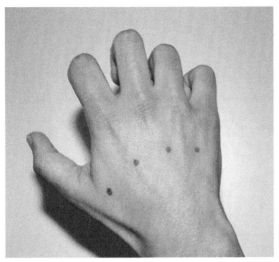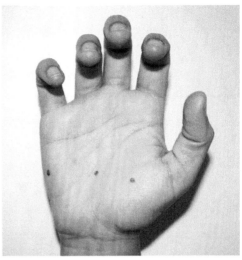

Fig. 5. Dorsal and volar views of hand with markings depicting potential interstitial pressure measurement sites.

released, and necrotic tissue is removed. Skin is usually left open and closed secondarily, skin grafted, or allowed to heal by secondary intention when swelling has resolved. The interosseous compartments can be released with 2 dorsal incisions, one between the index and long metacarpals and the other between the ring and small finger metacarpals, avoiding surgical wounds directly over the extensors to avoid tendon desiccation. Dissecting and releasing the investing fascia on either side of the metacarpals will decompress the dorsal interossei. Deeper dissection releases the palmar interossei. The first dorsal interosseous and adductor pollicis are released by dissecting radially along the index metacarpal (Fig. 6).[34]

Volar incisions can be made to release the thenar and hypothenar compartments along the glabrous–nonglabrous skin junction. For the thenar compartment, an incision along the radial thumb metacarpal border can be used. The hypothenar incision is made along the ulnar border of the small finger metacarpal (Fig. 7).

The carpal canal is decompressed with a separate volar approach that has been well-described and extends in the axis of the ring finger, in the interthenar cleft extending proximally from Kaplan's cardinal line. If there is concern for finger compartment syndrome from digital swelling, as often happens in burns, midaxial lateral incisions can be made, being mindful of the digital neurovascular bundles.

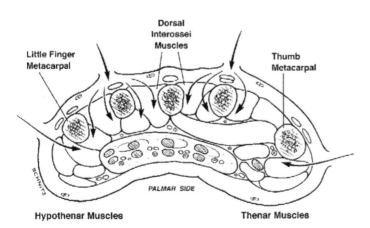

Fig. 6. Cross-sectional illustration of hand with arrows showing surgical access for compartment decompression. (*From* Seiler JG, Olvey SP. Compartment syndromes of the hand and forearm. J Am Soc Surg Hand 2003;3(4):186; with permission.)

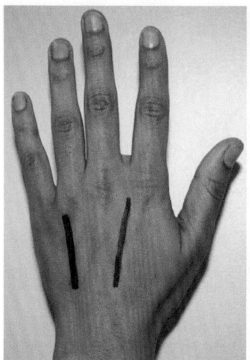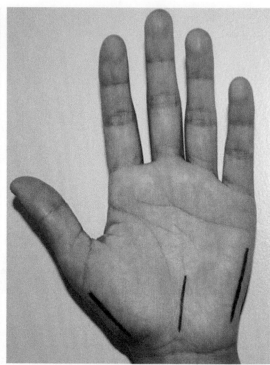

Fig. 7. Dorsal and volar views of hand with markings representing incision sites for hand compartment decompression surgery.

These are made along the ulnar aspect of the index, ring, and long fingers with radial sided incisions on the thumb and small fingers.[34]

Postoperative Management

The wounds are generally left open and covered with a sterile dressing or vacuum-assisted closure device. Serial explorations are indicated if there is concern about muscle viability. Wounds should be reevaluated every 2 to 3 days to continue debridement or perform delayed wound closure versus reconstruction when conditions permit. Teaming up with a hand therapist to facilitate range of motion exercises, edema control, wound care, and intrinsic plus splinting will minimize contractures and stiffness. If the skin is a concern and cannot be splinted, as in a patient with a burn, the metacarpophalangeal joints can be pinned in intrinsic plus. It is also important during postoperative therapy to range the proximal interphalangeal joints to avoid extension contractures.

Outcome data for isolated hand compartment syndrome are scarce. In lower extremity trauma, a shorter interval to fasciotomy, younger age, absence of bony injury or concomitant injuries, and low-velocity crush injuries tended to predict better outcomes.[42] In a systematic review of forearm compartment syndrome, neurologic deficit was the most common complication (21%).[43] In a retrospective review in children, compartment syndrome cases were grouped (forearm and hand) with excellent long-term outcomes in 17 (74%) and fair in 5 (22%) based on motor function, stiffness, or decreased sensation.[44] Ouellette and Kelly[8] reported 13 of 17 patients with normal hand function at average 21 month follow-up (2 of which had required secondary procedure for release of hand contractures), 4 patients had poor results with time from compartment syndrome recognition to fasciotomy exceeding 6 hours. In general, delays in diagnosis and worsening injury severity, with muscle or nerve damage, can result in inferior functional outcomes.

SUMMARY

Hand compartment syndrome has many etiologies and severe consequences if untreated. The pathophysiology involves the increase of pressures within an osteofascial compartment causing decreased tissue perfusion and leading to progressive muscle and soft tissue death. Clinical findings can evolve over time, so serial examinations and, if necessary, interstitial pressure monitoring are critical in expeditious diagnosis. Early recognition and compartment release is crucial to avoid tissue damage and preserve hand function.

REFERENCES

1. Amsdell SL, Hammert WC. High-pressure injection injuries in the hand. Plast Reconstr Surg 2013; 132(4):586e–91e.
2. Cohen J, Bush S. Case report: compartment syndrome after a suspected black widow spider bite. Ann Emerg Med 2005;45(4):414–6.
3. Cosker T, Gupta S, Tayton K. Compartment syndrome caused by suction. Injury 2004;35(11):1194–5.
4. Funk L, Grover D, de Silva H. Compartment syndrome of the hand following intra-arterial injection of heroin. J Hand Surg Am 1999;24(3): 366–7.
5. Abdul-Hamid AK. First dorsal interosseous compartment syndrome. J Hand Surg Br 1987; 12(2):269–72.
6. Hung LK, Kinninmonth AW, Woo ML. Vibrio vulnificus necrotizing fasciitis presenting with compartmental syndrome of the hand. J Hand Surg Am 1988;13(3):337–9.
7. Jensen SL, Sandermann J. Compartment syndrome and fasciotomy in vascular surgery. A review of 57 cases. Eur J Vasc Endovasc Surg 1997; 13(1):48–53.
8. Ouellette EA, Kelly R. Compartment syndromes of the hand. J Bone Joint Surg Am 1996;78(10): 1515–22.
9. Sawyer JR, Kellum EL, Creek AT, et al. Acute compartment syndrome of the hand after a wasp sting: a case report. J Pediatr Orthop B 2010; 19(1):82–5.
10. Selek H, Özer H, Aygencel G, et al. Compartment syndrome in the hand due to extravasation of contrast material. Arch Orthop Trauma Surg 2007; 127(6):425–7.
11. Shin AY, Chambers H, Wilkins KE, et al. Suction injuries in children leading to acute compartment syndrome of the interosseous muscles of the hand: case reports. J Hand Surg Am 1996;21(4): 675–8.
12. Tosti R, Ilyas AM. Acute carpal tunnel syndrome. Orthop Clin North Am 2012;43(4):459–65.
13. Matsen FA 3rd. Compartmental syndrome. An unified concept. Clin Orthop Relat Res 1975;(113):8–14.
14. Dahlin LB, Rydevik B, McLean WG, et al. Changes in fast axonal transport during experimental nerve compression at low pressures. Exp Neurol 1984; 84(1):29–36.
15. Matava MJ, Whitesides TEJ, Seiler JG 3rd, et al. Determination of the compartment pressure threshold of muscle ischemia in a canine model. J Trauma 1994;37(1):50–8.
16. Hargens AR, Mubarak SJ. Current concepts in the pathophysiology, evaluation, and diagnosis of compartment syndrome. Hand Clin 1998;14(3): 371–83.
17. Gelberman RH, Szabo RM, Williamson RV, et al. Tissue pressure threshold for peripheral nerve viability. Clin Orthop Relat Res 1983;178: 285–91.
18. Hargens AR, Botte MJ, Swenson MR, et al. Effects of local compression on peroneal nerve function in humans. J Orthop Res 1993;11(6): 818–27.
19. Heckman MM, Whitesides TEJ, Grewe SR, et al. Histologic determination of the ischemic threshold of muscle in the canine compartment syndrome model. J Orthop Trauma 1993;7(3):199–210.
20. Whitesides TE, Heckman MM. Acute compartment syndrome: update on diagnosis and treatment. J Am Acad Orthop Surg 1996;4(4):209–18.
21. Zandi H, Bell S. Results of compartment decompression in chronic forearm compartment syndrome: six case presentations. Br J Sports Med 2005;39(9):e35.
22. Ardolino A, Zeineh N, O'Connor D. Experimental study of forearm compartmental pressures. J Hand Surg Am 2010;35(10):1620–5.
23. Seiler JG 3rd, Womack S, De L'Aune WR, et al. Intracompartmental pressure measurements in the normal forearm. J Orthop Trauma 1993;7(5): 414–6.
24. Heppenstall RB, Sapega AA, Scott R, et al. The compartment syndrome. An experimental and clinical study of muscular energy metabolism using phosphorus nuclear magnetic resonance spectroscopy. Clin Orthop Relat Res 1988;(226): 138–55.
25. Mubarak SJ, Hargens AR. Acute compartment syndromes. Surg Clin North Am 1983;63(3):539–65.
26. Whitesides TE, Haney TC, Morimoto K, et al. Tissue pressure measurements as a determinant for the need of fasciotomy. Clin Orthop Relat Res 1975;(113):43–51.
27. Codding JL, Vosbikian MM, Ilyas AM. Acute compartment syndrome of the hand. J Hand Surg Am 2015;40(6):1213–6.
28. Lipschitz AH, Lifchez SD. Measurement of compartment pressures in the hand and forearm. J Hand Surg Am 2010;35(11):1893–4.
29. Chandraprakasam T, Kumar RA. Acute compartment syndrome of forearm and hand. Indian J Plast Surg 2011;44(2):212–8.
30. Leversedge FJ, Moore TJ, Peterson BC, et al. Compartment syndrome of the upper extremity. J Hand Surg Am 2011;36(3):544–59.
31. Difelice A, Gray J, Iii S, et al. The compartments of the hand: an anatomic study. J Hand Surg Am 1998;23:682–6.

32. Guyton GP, Shearman CM, Saltzman CL. Compartmental divisions of the hand revisited. Rethinking the validity of cadaver infusion experiments. J Bone Joint Surg Br 2001;83(2):241–4.

33. Ling MZX, Kumar VP. Myofascial compartments of the hand in relation to compartment syndrome: a cadaveric study. Plast Reconstr Surg 2009;123(2): 613–6.

34. Seiler JG, Olvey SP. Compartment syndromes of the hand and forearm. J Am Soc Surg Hand 2003; 3(4):184–98.

35. Duckworth AD, Mitchell SE, Molyneux SG, et al. Acute compartment syndrome of the forearm. J Bone Joint Surg Am 2012;94(10):e63.

36. Griffiths DL. Volkmann's ischaemic contracture. Br J Surg 1940;28(110):239–60.

37. Matsen FA 3rd, Mayo KA, Sheridan GW, et al. Monitoring of intramuscular pressure. Surgery 1976;79(6):702–9.

38. Mubarak SJ, Hargens AR, Owen CA, et al. The wick catheter technique for measurement of intramuscular pressure. A new research and clinical tool. J Bone Joint Surg Am 1976;58(7):1016–20.

39. Rorabeck CH, Castle GS, Hardie R, et al. Compartmental pressure measurements: an experimental investigation using the slit catheter. J Trauma 1981;21(6):446–9.

40. Wong JC, Vosbikian MM, Dwyer JM, et al. Accuracy of measurement of hand compartment pressures: a cadaveric study. J Hand Surg Am 2015; 40(4):701–6.

41. Daniels M, Reichman J, Brezis M. Mannitol treatment for acute compartment syndrome. Nephron 1998;79(4):492–3.

42. Han F, Daruwalla ZJ, Shen L, et al. A prospective study of surgical outcomes and quality of life in severe foot trauma and associated compartment syndrome after fasciotomy. J Foot Ankle Surg 2015; 54(3):417–23.

43. Kalyani BS, Fisher BE, Roberts CS, et al. Compartment syndrome of the forearm: a systematic review. J Hand Surg Am 2011;36(3):535–43.

44. Kanj WW, Gunderson MA, Carrigan RB, et al. Acute compartment syndrome of the upper extremity in children: diagnosis, management, and outcomes. J Child Orthop 2013;7(3):225–33.

High-pressure Injection Injuries of the Hand

Tyler A. Cannon, MD*

KEYWORDS

• Injection • Pressure • Amputation • Ischemia • Debridement

KEY POINTS

- High-pressure injection injuries of the hand are often overlooked injuries with potentially devastating consequences and high rates of amputation.
- High-pressure injection injuries require broad-spectrum antibiotics, tetanus prophylaxis, and emergent surgical debridement and decompression within 6 hours of injury.
- Prognosis depends on the type of material involved, location, pressure, and time to surgical intervention.
- Frequent residual sequelae include stiffness, pain, sensation loss, and difficulties in returning to work.

INTRODUCTION

Injection injuries to the hand are uncommon and may have devastating consequences owing to the associated high pressure and serious risks. Initial presentation of high-pressure injection injuries to the hand may be deceptively benign. Small skin wounds with minimal discomfort or loss of function may suggest an innocuous injury; however, progressive swelling and pressure leads to severe pain, increasing pressure, and ultimately an ischemic digit with high amputation rates.[1] Failure to recognize and emergently treat high-pressure injection injuries to the hand leads to permanent and ultimately high rates of amputation.[2]

Historically, injection injuries have been noted to cause severe soft tissue injury with increased rates of amputation. Rees[3] in 1937 noted gangrene owing to injection of oil under high pressure that required ultimately amputation. In 1938, Dial[4] supported the severe nature of oil-based injection injuries to the hand. High-pressure injuries to the hand have continued to increase in numbers owing to the progressive industrialization of the economy.

EPIDEMIOLOGY

On average, 1 in 600 traumatic hand injuries involve a high-pressure injection injury, and large surgical centers average 1 to 4 injection injuries annually.[1] High-pressure injection injuries to the hand typically occur on the dominant hand, particularly the index finger. The majority of patients are male, manual laborers with a large percentage involving worker's compensation claims[5] (Table 1). Hogan and Ruland[6] found the nondominant extremity to be injured 78% of the time, and the index finger as the most common site of injury, followed by the middle finger and palm (Table 2). The most common scenario occurs at the workplace as the patient is an industrial worker who typically is accidentally injured from attempting to clean a nozzle with their nondominant hand. Often, many of these injuries involve an employee of a new job or handling unfamiliar equipment.[7] The majority of these injuries are first regarded as benign but quickly escalate to emergencies owing to intense pain from progressing pressure and edema formation.

The author has nothing to disclose.
Tabor Orthopedics, 1244 Primacy Parkway, Memphis, TN 38117, USA
* 1244 Primacy Parkway, Memphis, TN 38117.
E-mail address: bluecannon15@gmail.com

Orthop Clin N Am 47 (2016) 617–624
http://dx.doi.org/10.1016/j.ocl.2016.03.007
0030-5898/16/$ – see front matter © 2016 Elsevier Inc. All rights reserved.

Table 1
Demographic data of the occupational hand injured patients (n = 140)

Risk Factors	n	%
Gender		
Male	99	70.7
Female	41	29.3
Marital status		
Unmarried	50	35.7
Married	85	60.7
Other[a]	5	3.6
Salary level (NTD[b][c])		
<20,000	35	30.4
20,000–30,000	37	32.2
≥30,001	43	37.4
Education level (y)		
<10	48	34.3
10–12	54	38.6
≥13	38	27.1
Occupation		
White collar	45	32.1
Blue collar	95	67.9
Workers' compensation		
No	38	27.1
Yes	102	72.9
Age (y)		Mean ± SD
	140	42.6 ± 12.9

[a] Other marital status includes separation and divorce.
[b] 33 NTD (New Taiwan Dollar) = 1 USD.
[c] Numbers of subjects do not add up to total n because of missing data.

From Lee Y, Chang J, Shieh S, et al. Association between the initial anatomical severity and opportunity of return to work in occupational hand injured patients. J Trauma 2010;69:E88–93; with permission.

PATHOPHYSIOLOGY

After high-pressure injections injuries, rapid development of tissue necrosis occurs from the inciting pressure. Injected materials themselves may be caustic and directly injure the surrounding soft tissue to further produce additional necrosis and significant damage to the surrounding tissues. An acute inflammatory reaction follows, causing elevated fluid pressures within confined compartment volumes. The increased compartmental pressures then cause vasospasm, leading to further swelling, local

Table 2
Most common locations of high-pressure injection injuries to the upper extremity

Location	n
Index	172
Long	64
Ring	20
Small	6
Thumb	41
Palm	62
"Hand" or "finger"	16
Forearm	7

From Hogan CJ, Ruland RT. High-pressure injection injuries to the upper extremity: a review of the literature. J Orthop Trauma 2006;20(7):504; with permission.

ischemia, and thrombosis. The result of this ever-increasing inflammatory response is a vicious cycle of swelling, ischemia, and ultimately compartment syndrome. Without acute and emergent operative intervention, ischemia ensues and the loss of the digit may be inevitable.

PROGNOSIS
Injected Material

The composition of the injected material is important as many of the components amplify the inflammatory response from direct toxicity causing further tissue necrosis. Grease, diesel fuel, and paint are some of the most common injected substances, and paint is associated with a particularly poor outcome.[8]

In a study of 127 patients with high-pressure injections, Schoo and colleagues[9] determined an average amputation rate of 48% (Table 3).

Table 3
Incidence of amputation (average, 48%)

Material	No. of Patients	No. of Patients with Amputations	Percentage
Paint thinner	5	4	80
Diesel fuel	6	4	67
Paint	36	21	58
Grease	40	9	23
Hydraulic fluid	7	1	14

From Schoo MJ, Scott FA, Boswick JA Jr. High-pressure injection injuries of the hand. J Trauma 1980;20(3):243; with permission.

The highest incidence of amputation from high-pressure injections was at 80% owing to paint thinner, followed by 67% from diesel fuel injections and 58% from paint injections. Grease injections are less inflammatory and had much lower amputation rates. Grease has a tendency to produce chronic granulomas rather than direct chemical irritation.[10]

Hogan and colleagues later reported from a study of 435 patients that organic solvents are the agents with the highest rates of amputation (**Fig. 1**). The worst outcomes from high-pressure injections involved diesel, followed by paint thinner and oil. High-pressure injections of air or water had the most favorable outcomes and did not result in amputation, likely owing to the innocuous nature of these materials. Paint is composed of multiple components, each classified into 1 of 4 main categories: a binder, solvent, pigment, and additive.[9] Oil-based paints have a much greater risk for amputation (58%) compared with latex-based paints (6%).[6] Each of these categories injure the soft tissues directly and create a higher inflammatory response owing to their cytotoxic nature.

Other materials have also been described in the literature, such as cement,[11,12] hydrochloric acid,[13] dry cleaning solvents,[14] insecticides,[15] natural gas,[16] silicone,[17] and vaccinations.[18,19]

As a chemical irritant promoting further necrosis and inflammation, materials from the majority of high-pressure injections of the hand must be completely removed to stop the inflammatory response, ultimately leading to ischemia of the digit. Rare high-pressure injections of water, air, and small volume vaccinations may be treated initially with observation, and successful results have been reported without operative intervention.[20]

Location

The location of high-pressure injections impacts the prognosis and rate of amputation. Owing to limited space and volume, injections toward the fingertips typically involve higher rates of amputations than more proximal locations, such as the palm or thumb.[10] The injected material tends to spread by following the paths of least resistance, typically the neurovascular bundles and flexor tendon sheaths.[21,22] Injections within the thumb and small finger may spread proximally via the radial and ulnar bursa, respectively, to the forearm and even more proximal locations, whereas injections within the index, middle, and long fingers tend not to spread proximally and may be associated with higher amputation rates owing to higher accumulation of pressure. Hogan and Ruland[6] have shown a 69% amputation rate with injections of caustic materials to the fingers, an amputation rate 3 times greater than that of caustic material injected to the thumb and small finger. Remote spread after injections has been reported, with 1 case citing pneumomediastinum from an air gun injury to the hypothenar space that traveled along the ulnar artery.[23,24]

Pressure

Pressures as low as 100 psi are sufficient to penetrate the skin,[7] and working pressures may be as high as 10,000 psi. The higher the pressure and greater the volume of injected material, the greater the damage and extent of injury will be for the patient. Many injections occur from

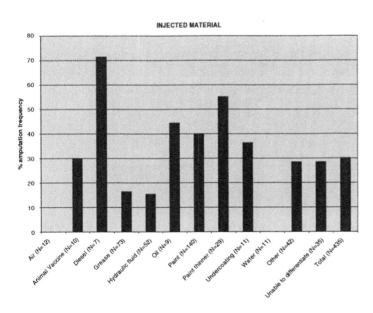

INJECTED MATERIAL

Fig. 1. Most commonly injected materials and associated risks of amputation. (*From* Hogan CJ, Ruland RT. High-pressure injection injuries to the upper extremity: a review of the literature. J Orthop Trauma 2006;20(7):504; with permission.)

placing the finger or thumb over the nozzle, causing even high amounts of pressure to be injected to the hand. Injections of greater than 1000 psi resulted in amputation 43% of the time, and injections of less than 1000 psi had amputation rates at 19% of the time.[6]

Timing

Perhaps the most important factor for physicians treating high-pressure injections is time of injury to surgical intervention, because time to operation is the 1 factor within the surgeon's control for treatment of these devastating injuries. Emergent operative intervention is warranted for high-pressure injuries other than potentially air and water to decompress the progressing pressure as well as to prevent and remove the toxicity to the surrounding tissues caused by the offending agent.[25]

The timing of thorough decompression and debridement has been directly associated with lowering the risk of amputation for organic high-pressure injections of organic solvents (paint, paint thinner, gasoline, oil, or jet fuel).[6] Debridement within 6 hours of high-pressure organic solvent injections has significantly lowered the amputation rate to 40% of the time, compared with an amputation rate of 57% if debridement was delayed for longer than 6 hours. Amputation rates of 88% are found if debridement is delayed for longer than 1 week.[6] Likely owing to the less toxic nature and lower amputation rates of materials not classified as organic solvents, Hogan and Ruland[6] did not find time to debridement to be a significant factor for treatment of more benign injected materials.

Patient Evaluation Overview

The course of high-pressure injection injuries usually begins with a small, innocuous-appearing entry wound that many times is overlooked[6] (Fig. 2A). The initial clinical appearance is typical underestimated; however, within hours, pain progressively intensifies and parallels marked swelling and edema of the affected extremity (Fig. 2B). The digit may quickly become cold, pale, and erythematous with associated paresthesia. Without prompt treatment, gangrene and sepsis may quickly follow.[26] Radiographs may be helpful to not only determine the location of the radiopaque foreign body and air, but also to reveal the dispersal of injected material proximally.[20] Emergent surgical decompression and debridement is the mainstay for most high-pressure injections.

TREATMENT

Initial treatment involves that all high-pressure injection injuries require broad-spectrum antibiotic (typically a first- or third-generation cephalosporin or gentamycin) and tetanus toxoid.[2,27,28] Hot soaks have also been shown to be detrimental to success rates after high-pressure injection injuries owing to further

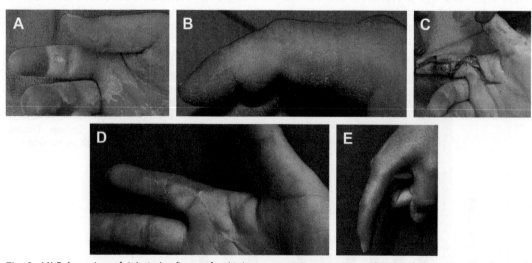

Fig. 2. (A) Palmer view of right index finger after high-pressure injection injury with paint thinner. Note small wound with paint thinner at base of wound and associated pallor throughout finger. (B) Lateral view of right index finger after high-pressure injection with paint thinner. Significant swelling and pallor along index finger in semiflexed position. (C) Palmer view of right index finger after decompression and debridement of right index finger. Return of blood flow demonstrated. Wound left open without formal closure, and immediate range of motion begun after surgery. (D, E) Final follow-up picture postoperative showing healed wound and functional range of motion.

exacerbation of the inflammatory response.[2] Use of steroids is controversial. Phelps and colleagues[29] showed a potential beneficial role of steroids to minimize small vessel thrombosis through the reduction inflammation and edema. No significant risk of infection has been associated with use of systemic steroids.[29] Despite the theoretic benefits to steroid treatment, no significant impact from the use of steroids has been seen concerning the prevention of amputation.[6]

Nonsurgical Treatment

Nonsurgical treatment for high-pressure injuries is rare but in some cases justified. High-pressure water injuries may be watched initially with a high clinical suspicion if edema and pain are reasonably controlled owing to the nontoxic nature of the injected material.[30] Injections of air and small veterinary vaccines similarly may also be treated with intravenous antibiotics and very close observation.[6,20] In either case, if pain and edema progress, emergent decompression and fasciotomy are required for impending compartment syndrome.[20] Although some authors have had success with initial high-pressured injections to the palm, this conservative treatment is debatable and most injection injuries to the palm require debridement and decompression.[31]

Surgical Treatment

Surgical treatment consists of decompression, wide debridement, and removal of injected material (Fig. 2C). Use of a tourniquet has been found to be safe; however, Esmarch exsanguination is discouraged because it may contribute to the proximal spread of injected material. Local anesthetic infiltration as well as Bier block is not recommended because these techniques may add further damage from increased pressure within the zone of injury.[20] Boyes cautioned against local digital block to avoid any additional measures that may increase swelling and vasospasm in the fingers.[32] General or regional anesthesia is preferred for wide surgical debridement, which may need to be extended proximally owing to spread of material. Decompression of fascial compartments is performed to relieve associated pressure, vasospasm, and ischemia. The digital neurovascular bundles and flexor tendon sheaths are explored because these are the primary means of foreign body proximal spread.[14,22,33] Meticulous debridement and removal of as much foreign material as possible is essential and must be performed thoroughly

with complete removal of all contaminated tissue because the injected material itself causes the soft tissue reaction and saline lavage does not remove insoluble materials such as oil-based paint.[25] Use of microsurgical techniques for removal of paint and other caustic agents is helpful and often performed and to avoid further damage to the neurovascular bundles.

After thorough debridement and decompression has been performed, repeat debridements within 48 to 72 hours often are necessary as "second-look" procedures, which serve several purposes. Second washouts are frequently necessary to remove any additional remaining foreign body or necrotic tissue. This time also is vital in determining viability of the digit, need for amputation, and possible closure procedures.[27,34]

The most effective means of closure is debatable. Pinto and colleagues[35] achieved a low amputation rate of 16% with open wound packing. Wound vacuum-assisted closure,[36] heterodigital island flaps,[37] cross-finger flaps,[38] and free toe pulp transfer[39] have also been described.

RESULTS AND COMPLICATIONS
Motion

After decompression and debridement, stiffness is a major concern postoperatively. Compared with the contralateral uninjured hand, range of motion deficits after high-pressure injection injuries to the hand averaged 8° at the metacarpophalangeal joint, 24° at the proximal interphalangeal joint, and 30° at the distal interphalangeal joint.[40] Immediate range of motion and initiation of hand therapy is critical for optimal postoperative success, and motion is usually begun postoperatively without restrictions (Fig. 2D, E).

Strength and Sensation

After high-pressure injection injuries and subsequent debridement, some sensation loss and weakness is usually expected. Wieder and colleagues[40] have shown average reductions in grip strength by 19%, key pinch by 23%, and 3-point pinch by 25%. Only 8% of patients had normal sensation, 58% light touch, 255 diminished protective sensation, and 8% lost protective sensation.[41] An average difference of 2-point discrimination from injured to noninjured hand was 49%. Given the extensive necrosis and ensuing scar formation, patients can anticipate at least mild to moderate loss of strength and sensation after successful debridement of high-pressure injection injuries to the hand.

Return to Work

Return to work averaged 7.5 months after injury. Only 44% of patients returned to their previous occupation; 39% of patients were employed at a different job and 17% remained unemployed.[40] The ability to return to work depends on many factors, including gender, education level, occupation, age, worker's compensation, and salary; however, possibly the most significant factor for return to work is the severity of injury.[5] Associated motor and, most important, neural deficits had the most negative influence on return to work status, and pain secondary to neural or motor loss was most responsible for lack of return to work. Nerve injury also leads to longer recovery times and patients with previous higher salaries had a high percentage of return to work than lower salary paid patients. Owing to long recovery times from severe injuries encountered after high-pressure injections, patients may expect prolonged time off before returning to work. Fewer than one-half of patients will resume their previous position, and almost 20% of patients will remain unemployed.

Retained Foreign Body

Incomplete debridement may lead to further complications, including formations of oleogranulomas, foreign body granulomas, and fibrohistiocytic tumors.[42] Chronic sinus tract formation may be present requiring additional operative intervention.[43] Of the most common injected materials, grease is a known substance with a high risk of granuloma formation.[10] Complete remove all foreign material is extremely difficult but should be the initial surgical goal to prevent such potential complications and additional surgeries.

Secondary Infection

Although many injected substances possess antibacterial properties, high-pressure injection injuries of foreign material within the extremity do involve a substantial risk for infection given the severe soft tissue inflammation and necrosis. Up to 41% of intraoperative cultures on initial debridement after injection injuries are positive, with many of these patients showing polymicrobial organisms. The presence of infection, however, did not affect the amputation rate.[6] Multiple studies advocate the use of broad-spectrum antibiotics given the high chance of infection.

Table 4 Subjective patient complaints after high-pressure injections to the hand	
Patient Complaint	Percentage of Patients
Cold intolerance	78
Hypersensitivity	61
Paresthesia	35
Constant pain	22
Impaired daily activities	22

From Wieder A, Lapid O, Plakht Y, et al. Long-term follow-up of high-pressure injection injuries to the hand. Plast Reconstr Surg 2006;117(1):188; with permission.

OTHER CONSIDERATIONS

Patients carried with them multiple other complaints after high-pressure injection injuries to the hand. The majority of patients complained of cold intolerance (78%) and hypersensitivity at the injection site (61%). Other less common issues included residual paresthesia (35%), constant pain (22%), and impaired activities (22%; Table 4). After the injection injury and subsequent debridement, many patients were left with visible scars (91%), deformed digits (86%), and other aesthetic complaints (Table 5). High-pressure injection injuries to the hand cause significant and often permanent sequelae that may impair function and daily activities.

Table 5 Objective patient complaints after surgical debridement for high-pressure injection injuries to the hand	
Visual Complaint	Percentage of Patients
Visible scar	91
Deformation of finger shape	86
Nail deformity	29
Amputation	22
Contracture	13
Residual paint	9

From Wieder A, Lapid O, Plakht Y, et al. Long-term follow-up of high-pressure injection injuries to the hand. Plast Reconstr Surg 2006;117(1):188; with permission.

SUMMARY

High-pressure injection injuries to the hand are often overlooked injuries with severe complications owing to the acute inflammatory response resulting from accumulating pressure, direct toxicity of the injected material, and progressive ischemia. The prognosis for the successful salvage of the digit depends on the type of material injected, location of injection, involved pressure, and, most important, timing to surgical decompression and debridement. Essential to successful outcome and the survival of the digit, acute management of high-pressure injection injuries involve broad-spectrum antibiotics, tetanus prophylaxis, and typically emergent decompression of all involved fascial compartments and complete removal with microsurgical technique of injected material. Most patients have residual and permanent sequelae. Stiffness, pain, sensation loss, and difficulties in return to work are not unusual for the majority of patients after high-pressure injection injuries to the hand. The hand surgeon's role in treating most patients with high-pressure injection injuries is prompt surgical intervention within 6 hours from injury, early motion and therapy, education of the patient regarding short and long-term expectations, and education of the emergency room staff and primary care providers. Preventative measures need to be emphasized and performed to avert such injuries from occurring.[44]

REFERENCES

1. Verhoeven N, Hierner R. High-pressure injection injury of the hand: An often underestimated trauma. Case report with study of the literature. Strategies Trauma Limb Reconstr 2008;3(1):27–33.

2. O'Reilly RJ, Blatt G. Accidental high pressure injection gun injuries of the hand. J Trauma 1975;15:24–31.

3. Rees CE. Penetration of tissue by fuel oil under high pressure from diesel engine. J Am Med Assoc 1937;109:866–7.

4. Dial DE. Hand injuries due to injection of oil at high pressures. J Am Med Assoc 1938;110:1747.

5. Lee Y, Chang J, Shieh S, et al. Association between the initial anatomical severity and opportunity of return to work in occupational hand injured patients. J Trauma 2010;69:E88–93.

6. Hogan CJ, Ruland RT. High-pressure injection injuries to the upper extremity: a review of the literature. J Orthop Trauma 2006;20(7):503–11.

7. Mills C, Wilson P, Watts T, et al. High pressure paint injection injury of the hand. Inj Extra 2007; 38:298–300.

8. Gelberman RH, Posch JL, Jurist JM. High-pressure injection injuries of the hand. J Bone Joint Surg Am 1975;57:935–7.

9. Schoo MJ, Scott FA, Boswick JA Jr. High-pressure injection injuries of the hand. J Trauma 1980;20(3): 229–38.

10. Rosenwasser MP, Wei DH. High-pressure Injection Injuries to the Hand. J Am Acad Orthop Surg 2014;22:38–45.

11. Barr ST, Wittenborn W, Nguyen D, et al. High-pressure cement injection injury of the hand: a case report. J Hand Surg 2002;27A:347.

12. Hutchinson CH. Hand injuries caused by injection of cement under pressure. J Bone Joint Surg Br 1968;50-B:131–3.

13. Bucklew PS, Horner WR, Diamond DL. High-pressure acid injection: case report with recommended initial management and therapy. J Trauma 1985; 25(6):552–6.

14. Gutowski KA, Chu J, Choi M, et al. High-pressure hand injection injuries caused by dry cleaning solvents: case reports, review of the literature, and treatment guidelines. Plast Reconstr Surg 2003;111(1):174–7.

15. Buchman MT. Upper extremity injection of household insecticide: a report of five cases. J Hand Surg 2000;25A:764.

16. Sena T, Brewer BW. Natural gas inflation injury of the upper extremity: a case report. J Hand Surg 1999;24A:850–2.

17. Apfelberg DB, Lash H, Maser MR, et al. High-pressure silicone injection injury of the hand. J Trauma 1975;15(10):922–5.

18. Couzens G, Burke FD. Veterinary high pressure injection injuries with inoculations for larger animals. J Hand Surg Br 1995;20(4):497–9.

19. Neal NC, Burke FD. High-pressure injection injuries. Injury 1991;22(6):467–70.

20. Amsdell SL, Hammert WC. High-pressure injection injuries in the hand: current treatment concepts. Plast Reconstr Surg 2013;132(4):586e–91e.

21. Ramos H, Posch JL, Lie KK. High pressure injection injuries of the hand. Plast Reconstr Surg 1970;45(3): 221–6.

22. Kaufman HD. The anatomy of experimentally produced high-pressure injection injuries of the hand. Br J Surg 1968;55(5):340–4.

23. Temple CL, Richards RS, Dawson WB. Pneumomediastinum after injection injury to the hand. Ann Plast Surg 2000;45(1):64–6.

24. Steffen T, Wedel A, Kluckert JT, et al. Severe pneumomediastinum after high-pressure air-injection injury to the hand: a case of pneumomediastinum with an unusual cause. J Trauma 2009;66:1243–5.

25. Failla JM, Linden MD. The acute pathologic changes of paint injection injury and correlation

to surgical treatment: a report of two cases. J Hand Surg Am 1997;22A:156–9.

26. Mann RJ. Paint and grease gun injuries of the hand. JAMA 1975;231:933.

27. Pappou IP, Deal DN. High-pressure injection injuries. J Hand Surg 2012;37A:2404–7.

28. Mirzayan R, Schnall SB, Chon JH, et al. Culture results and amputation rates in high-pressure paint gun injuries of the hand. Orthopedics 2001;24(6):587–9.

29. Phelps DB, Hastings H, Boswick JA. Systemic corticosteroid therapy for high pressure injection injuries of the hand. J Trauma 1976;17:206–10.

30. Pai CH, Wei DC, Hou SP. High-pressure injection injuries of the hand. J Trauma 1991;31(1):110–2.

31. Kendrick RW, Colville J. Conservative management of a high pressure injection injury to the hand. Hand 1982;14:159.

32. Stark HH, Ashworth CR, Boyes JH. Paint-gun injuries of the hand. J Bone Joint Surg 1967;49A:637–47.

33. Lewis HG, Clarke P, Kneafsey B, et al. A 10-year review of high pressure injection injuries to the hand. J Hand Surg Br 1998;23(4):479–81.

34. Ştefănescu RL, Bordelanu I. High-pressure injection injury of the finger- a case presentation. Clujul Med 2013;86(1):74–6.

35. Pinto MR, Turkula-Pinto LD, Cooney WP, et al. High-pressure injection injuries of the hand: review of 25 patients managed by open wound technique. J Hand Surg Am 1993;18(1):125–30.

36. Chen Q, Liu DS, Hu W, et al. Treatment of high-pressure pain injection injuries of hand with debridement combined with vacuum sealing drainage technique. Zhongguo Gu Shang 2011;24:851–3 [in Chinese].

37. Beckler H, Gokce A, Beyzadeoglu T, et al. The surgical treatment and outcomes of high-pressure injection injuries of the hand. J Hand Surg 2007;32B:394–9.

38. Oktem F, Ocguder A, Altuntas N, et al. High-pressure paint gun injection injury of the hand: a case report. J Plast Reconstr Aesthet Surg 2009;62:e157–9.

39. Chan BK, Tham SK, Leung M. Free toe pulp transfer for digital reconstruction after high-pressure injection injury. J Hand Surg 1999;24B:534–8.

40. Wieder A, Lapid O, Plakht Y, et al. Long-term follow-up of high-pressure injection injuries to the hand. Plast Reconstr Surg 2006;117(1):186–9.

41. Christodoulou L, Melikyan EY, Woodbridge S, et al. Functional outcome of high-pressure injection injuries of the hand. J Trauma 2001;50(4):717–20.

42. Saadat P, Vadmal M. Fibrohistiocytic tumor of the hand after high-pressure paintgun injury: 2 case reports. J Hand Surg 2005;30A(2):404–8.

43. Geller ER, Gursel E. A Unique Case of High-Pressure Injection Injury of the Hand. J Trauma 1986;26(5):483–5.

44. Hart RG, Smith GD, Haq A. Prevention of high-pressure injection injuries to the hand. Am J Emerg Med 2006;24:73–6.

Foot and Ankle

Review of Talus Fractures and Surgical Timing

Benjamin J. Grear, MD*

KEYWORDS

- Talus fracture • Delayed fixation • Surgical timing

KEY POINTS

- This article gives special attention to the clinical literature that evaluates the timing of surgical management for displaced talus fractures.
- Despite surgical fixation, high complication rates accompany displaced talar fractures, creating significant patient morbidity.
- Contrary to historical recommendations, delayed fixation for displaced talar fractures produces satisfactory outcomes, suggesting displaced fractures do not necessitate emergent surgical treatment.

INTRODUCTION

As the osseous link between the foot and leg, the talus is essential for normal gait mechanics. It involves both the ankle and the subtalar joint complexes through multiple articular surfaces with the fibula, tibia, calcaneus, and navicular. The talus consists of 3 main sections (body, head, and neck) and 2 processes (lateral and posterior processes). The posterior process is composed of 2 tubercles (posteromedial and posterolateral tubercles). Articular cartilage covers more than 65% of the talar surface, and no tendon or muscle attachments originate from the talus.[1] With its many articulations, fractures frequently lead to posttraumatic arthrosis, and malunions alter mechanics, creating disability. The exta-articular surface allows for ligamentous and capsular attachments and entrance for the extraosseous blood supply.[1] Traveling through these limited soft tissue attachments, the extraosseous blood supply is at risk for injury, making the talus prone to osteonecrosis. Talar injuries cause significant patient morbidity, highlighting the importance of effective and efficient treatment to minimize resultant complications.

High-energy mechanisms such as falls from a height or motor vehicle accidents account for most fractures, but low-energy mechanisms, such as sports injuries, have also been reported.[2–4] Because of the distraction of other injuries in critically ill patients or the decreased awareness in unsuspecting sport injuries, talus fractures may be undiagnosed on initial presentation. Clinicians must maintain a high index of suspicion for any patient presenting with hindfoot pain after an acute injury. These patients should have a detailed history and physical examination plus dedicated foot and ankle radiographs, and any radiographic irregularities should prompt a computed tomographic (CT) scan to better identify and characterize talar fractures.

TALUS BLOOD SUPPLY

With osteonecrosis commonly reported as a complication in talar injuries, the blood supply of the talus has been extensively researched. The extraosseous blood supply includes branches from the posterior tibial artery (artery of the tarsal canal, deltoid branches), branches from anterior tibial artery (dorsalis pedis

Disclosure Statement: The author has nothing to disclose.

Department of Orthopaedic Surgery and Biomedical Engineering, University of Tennessee-Campbell Clinic, Memphis, TN, USA

* Campbell Clinic, 1400 South Germantown Road, Germantown, TN 38138.

E-mail address: bgrear@campbellclinic.com

Orthop Clin N Am 47 (2016) 625–637
http://dx.doi.org/10.1016/j.ocl.2016.03.008
0030-5898/16/$ – see front matter © 2016 Elsevier Inc. All rights reserved.

branches), and branches from the peroneal artery (posterior tubercle branches, artery of tarsal sinus). The artery of the tarsal canal (branch of the posterior tibial artery) gives off the deltoid branches supplying the medial talar body. The artery of the tarsal canal continues distally to join the artery of the tarsal sinus (branch of the peroneal artery) forming an important anastomosis inferior to the talar. Branches from this anastomosis enter the inferior neck supplying a significant portion of the talar body. Dorsalis pedis branches (branch of the anterior tibial artery) enter the dorsal neck supplying most of the talar neck and a portion of the talar head. The talar head is further supplied from the artery of the tarsal canal (branch of the peroneal artery). Last, the posterior tubercle branches (branch of the peroneal artery) contribute to the posterior process (Fig. 1).[5–7]

FRACTURE CLASSIFICATION

The Orthopedic Trauma Association (OTA) has extensively classified talus fractures, in which the fractures are divided into head fractures (81-A), neck fractures (81-B), and body fractures (81-C). Included in the head fracture category, avulsion and process fractures also receive the 81-A designation. Talar neck fractures are further divided into nondisplaced fractures (81-B1), fractures with subtalar joint incongruity (81-B2), and fractures with subtalar and tibiotalar joint incongruity (81-B3). Body fractures are divided into talar dome fractures (81-C1), talar body fractures with subtalar joint involvement (B1-C2), and body fractures with subtalar and tibiotalar joint involvement (81-C3). Fractures of the talar head, neck, and body are further classified according to comminution.[8] Talar neck fractures are also commonly classified according to Hawkins,[4] which is further discussed with talar neck fractures.

TALAR HEAD FRACTURES

Talar head fractures are very uncommon, accounting for less than 10% of all talus fractures, and there is limited clinical research that assessed these fractures.[9–11] Compression and shear forces have been described as mechanisms for injury. Forefoot impaction forces along the medial column create compression fractures, and navicular shear forces resultant from midfoot adduction create shear fractures to the medial talar head.[11] Radiographic evaluation should routinely involve anterior-to-posterior (AP), oblique, and lateral foot radiographs.

These fractures may be difficult to see on radiographs, particularly the plantar portion of the talar head. Any irregularities on radiographs should elicit advanced imaging.

The principles of treatment include maintenance of the medial column length and height, and restoring talonavicular joint congruity, stability, and motion. Nondisplaced fractures with a stable joint may be treated conservatively with immobilization and non-weight-bearing for 4 to 6 weeks,[9–13] but displaced fractures or joint instability requires operative treatment. Small comminuted fractures may be excised to restore talonavicular motion, but larger fragments are stabilized with headless screws, mini-fragment screws, or bioabsorbable implants (Fig. 2). Minimizing dorsal dissection, dorsal, or medial approaches are used depending on the fracture location. Unlike neck and body fractures, osteonecrosis is uncommon in talar head fractures, but posttraumatic arthritis is a likely complication following intra-articular fractures.

TALAR NECK FRACTURES

The area designated as the talar neck lies between the talar head and body (lateral process). This area is commonly injured, accounting for nearly half of all significant injuries to the talus.[4,9,10,13] Unlike most of the talus, the neck is void of articular cartilage, providing a site for soft tissue attachments and vascular foramen. Adjacent to the inferior talar neck, the artery of the tarsal canal joins the artery of the tarsal sinus forming an important anastomosis.[1,5–7] The close proximity of this anastomosis to the talar neck makes it vulnerable to injury with neck fractures, explaining the common complication of osteonecrosis.

As aforementioned, the OTA categorizes talar neck fractures according displacement and subtalar joint congruity,[8] but before the OTA classification, Hawkins classified talar neck fractures in 1970.[4] The Hawkins classification is still the most commonly used nomenclature to describe talar neck fractures. A Hawkins type I refers to a nondisplaced fracture of the talar neck. In a Hawkins type II, the neck fracture is accompanied by subtalar joint subluxation or dislocation. Type II fractures are the most common. Talar neck fractures with tibiotalar and subtalar incongruity represent Hawkins type III fractures. Last, Canale and Kelly[14] added the type IV modification, in which neck fractures are accompanied with complete talar dislocations (ie, tibiotalar, talonavicular, and subtalar joint incongruity) (Fig. 3). Osteonecrosis has been reported in type II fractures as high as

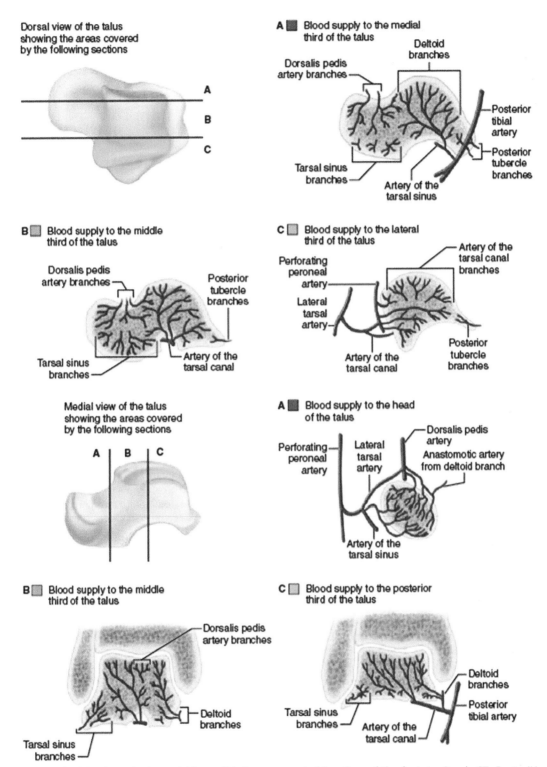

Fig. 1. Talar blood supply. (*From* Ishikawa SN. Fractures and dislocations of the foot. In: Canale ST, Beaty JH, editors. Campbell's operative orthopaedics. 12th edition. Philadelphia: Elsevier; 2013; with permission.)

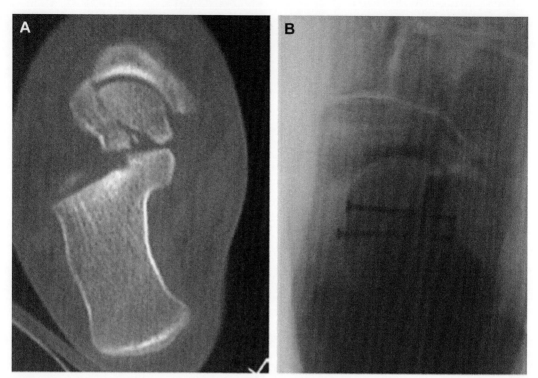

Fig. 2. (*A*) Displaced talar head fracture, (*B*) subsequent ORIF with mini-fragment lag screws. (*From* Early JS. Talus fracture management. Foot Ankle Clin N Am 2008;13(4):641; with permission.)

40% to 50%, and in type III and IV fractures as high as 100%.[14] Recently, Vallier and colleagues[3] suggested a modification of the Hawkins type II fracture, adding types IIA and IIB. In type IIA, the subtalar joint is mildly subluxated, and in type IIB, the subtalar joint is dislocated. Of 19 Hawkins type IIA fractures, none developed osteonecrosis, but 25% (4/16) of IIB fractures developed avascular necrosis (AVN).

For completely nondisplaced fractures (Hawkins type I), treatment consists of immobilization and non-weight-bearing for 6 weeks or until radiographic union.[4,15] If the fracture line is easily visible on radiographs, then the fracture should be appropriately classified as a Hawkins type II, and conservative treatment is not recommended. For any displaced neck fractures, anatomic reduction and rigid fixation are recommended. Complete joint dislocations require immediate closed reductions, but, as discussed separately, definitive fixation can be delayed.[3,16–18] Surgical approaches typically include dual incisions medially and laterally, but in simple, noncomminuted fractures, a percutaneous or single approach may be used. In addition, a posterolateral approach (open or percutaneous) may be added for posterior-to-anterior (PA) screw fixation (**Fig. 4**).

Fixation techniques include the use of small and mini-fragment lag screws (headed and headless) for noncomminuted fractures. With comminuted fractures, the surgeon should avoid fracture compression (ie, shortening malunion) by using length-preserving screw techniques or small plates.[19] Screws can be used in an AP or PA direction. PA screws generally provide fixation at an angle more perpendicular to the fracture line,[20] but PA screws also require additional exposure posterolaterally, adding increased dissection and difficulty in the supine position. With distal neck fractures, AP screws commonly require entrance through the talar head articular surface. By way of countersink techniques or headless implants, the talonavicular joint must remain free of hardware impingement (**Fig. 5**). Even with surgical treatment, complications include osteonecrosis, malunion, nonunion, and posttraumatic arthritis. Open injuries, displacement, and comminution negatively impact outcomes.[16,17]

TALAR BODY FRACTURES

Talar body fractures are defined as any fracture line at or posterior to the lateral tubercle of the talus.[21] Talar body fractures account for 7% to

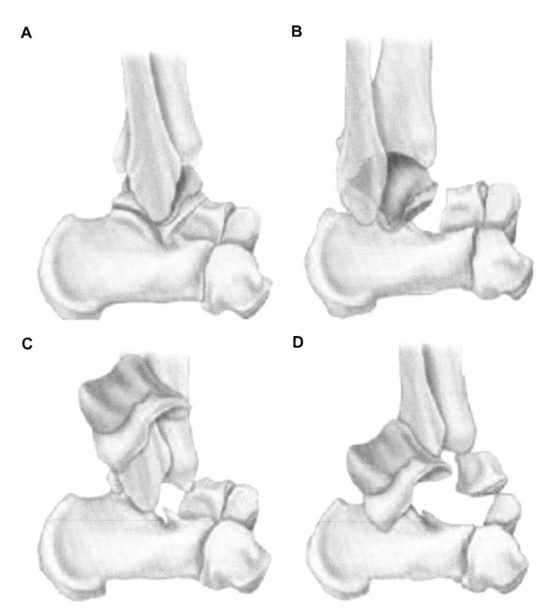

Fig. 3. Modified Hawkins classification. (*A*) Type I, (*B*) type II, (*C*) type III, (*D*) type IV. (*From* Ishikawa SN. Fractures and dislocations of the foot. In: Canale ST, Beaty JH, editors. Campbell's operative orthopaedics. 12th edition. Philadelphia: Elsevier; 2013; with permission.)

38% of all talar injuries.[11,22] The mechanism of injury typically involves high-energy compression between the tibial plafond and the calcaneus, but low-energy shearing forces can also generate body fractures. Corresponding with the high-energy mechanisms, open injuries are common, occurring in roughly 20% of body fractures.[23] Talar body fractures include lateral and posterior process fractures, which are discussed separately.

Treatment goals include restoration of stability and congruity for the tibiotalar and subtalar joints.

For displaced fractures, anatomic reduction and internal fixation are indicated. The reduction can be achieved through percutaneous, arthroscopic, or open approaches. A variety of approaches (lateral, medial, posterolateral, or posteromedial) may be used to achieve optimal visualization and reduction. Furthermore, medial or lateral malleoli osteotomies may be needed to visualize the talar dome reduction (**Fig. 6**). Despite surgical treatment, osteonecrosis, posttraumatic arthritis, and malunion are common sequelae.[23]

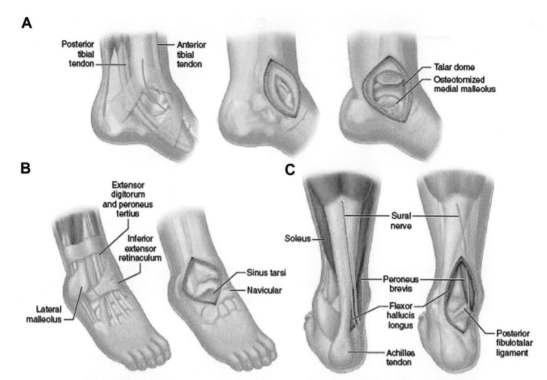

Fig. 4. (A) Medial approach, (B) lateral approach, (C) posterolateral approach. (*From* Ishikawa SN. Fractures and dislocations of the foot. In: Canale ST, Beaty JH, editors. Campbell's operative orthopaedics. 12th edition. Philadelphia: Elsevier; 2013; with permission.)

TIMING OF TREATMENT: ORTHOPEDIC EMERGENCY?

With the well-known vulnerability of the blood supply and the resultant osteonecrosis complications, investigators have historically recommended emergent treatment of displaced talus fractures.[4,14,15] However, more recent literature suggests that emergent open reduction internal fixation (ORIF) versus delayed ORIF has no significant difference in outcomes, making the timing of definitive fixation controversial.[3,16–18] Certainly, all open fractures should be treated emergently with debridement, irrigation, stabilization, and antibiotics, but definitive fixation may be delayed. Similarly, complete joint dislocations should undergo emergent reductions. If irreducible with closed techniques, then surgical reductions (percutaneous or open) should be performed emergently, but definitive fixation may be delayed. Theoretically, delaying fixation may even improve outcomes by allowing for soft tissue recovery before open surgical exposures, increasing time for enhanced surgical planning, and improving surgeon experience via appropriate transfers of care.

Lindvall and colleagues[18] retrospectively reviewed 26 displaced talar body and neck

fractures that underwent ORIF. A minimum of 48 months follow-up was required. The series consisted of 11 Hawkins type II fractures, 6 Hawkins type III fractures, 1 Hawkins type IV fracture, and 8 talar body fractures. Seven of the fractures were open injuries. The average follow-up was 73 months. Fractures treated within 6 hours after injury were compared with those that were treated after 6 hours. Twelve of the 26 fractures (46%) received surgical treatment within 6 hours. No significant difference in American Orthopaedic Foot and Ankle Society outcomes, nonunions, osteonecrosis, or posttraumatic arthritis was seen between fractures treated within 6 hours versus those fractures treated after 6 hours. The average time to surgery was 85 hours (range 2–504 hours). All displaced talar neck fractures healed regardless of time to surgery, including one that surgery was delayed for 21 days.

In another series, Sanders and colleagues[16] reviewed 70 displaced talar fractures. The investigators evaluated outcome scores and the need for secondary reconstructive surgery. Sixty-six patients underwent ORIF, whereas 4 required a talectomy due to gross contamination or loss at the scene. Fractures included 29 Hawkins

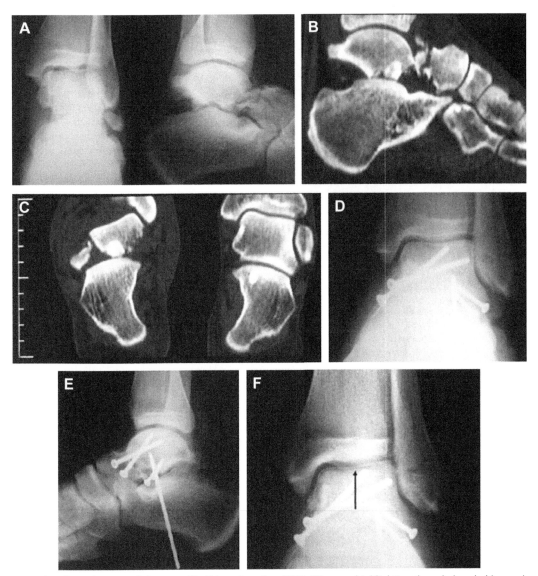

Fig. 5. (A–C) Hawkins type II fracture, (D, E) imaging after ORIF, (F) arrow highlighting the subchondral bone absorption (Hawkins sign). (From Rammelt S, Zwipp H. Talar neck and body fractures. Injury 2009;40:120; with permission.)

type II, 25 Hawkins type III, and 16 Hawkins type IV. Ten fractures were open injuries. The mean follow-up was 5.2 years. Twenty-six (37%) patients required a secondary reconstructive surgery, due to an absent talus (4), infection (5), malunion (5), arthrosis (11), and osteonecrosis (3). The time to surgery did not affect the need for secondary reconstructive procedures. However, the investigators did not list the detailed times in which surgery was performed, rendering the time from injury to surgery unknown. Patients were more likely to require secondary procedures for comminuted fractures and increased

displacement (ie, Hawkins type III or IV fractures).

Another group of investigators retrospectively reviewed 60 displaced talar neck fractures that required ORIF. Unfortunately, of these 60, only 39 had complete radiographic data. The average time from injury to definitive fixation was 3.7 days (range 4 hours to 48 days). Surgical fixation within 6 hours, 8 hours, 12 hours, 24 hours, or greater than 24 hours did not affect the osteonecrosis rate. Osteonecrosis occurred in 19 of 39 (49%). The mean time to fixation was 3.4 days (range, 4 hours to 20 days) for

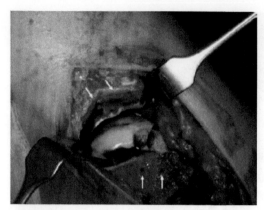

Fig. 6. Use of a medial malleolus osteotomy to visualize a talar dome fracture. The arrows indicate predrilled tunnels for later osteotomy fixation. (*From* Rammelt S, Zwipp H. Talar neck and body fractures. Injury 2009;40:120; with permission.)

those that developed osteonecrosis and 5.0 days (range, 4 hours to 48 days) for those that did not develop osteonecrosis. The amount of comminution and soft tissue injury (open fractures) significantly increased with the rate of osteonecrosis, and the amount of displacement (based on the Hawkins classification) showed a positive trend toward osteonecrosis.[17]

More recently, Vallier and colleagues retrospectively reviewed 81 talar neck fractures, of which 29 had concomitant talar body fractures. The cohort consisted of 2 Hawkins type I, 54 Hawkins type II, 32 Hawkins type III, and 3 Hawkins type IV. The investigators further categorized Hawkins type II fractures into those without subtalar joint dislocation (II-A) and those with subtalar dislocation (II-B). Twenty-one were type II-A, and 33 were type II-B.

Treatment consisted of emergent closed reduction in the emergency department for dislocation patterns. Irreducible dislocations and open fractures were taken to the operating room urgently. Otherwise, the timing and type of definitive fixation were at the surgeon's discretion. Nineteen (23%) were irreducible, and 22 (27%) were open fractures. At the surgeon's discretion, another 9 fractures were treated urgently, 4 of which had other injuries necessitating urgent operative treatment. In all, 46 (57%) were treated with urgent, definitive fixation. For those treated urgently, the mean time from injury to ORIF was 10.1 hours. The remaining 35 patients were treated with delayed ORIF. For the delayed group, the mean time from injury to ORIF was 10.6 days (range 3–19 days). In most patients, dual approaches with stainless steel small-fragment and/or mini-fragment implants were used. Patients remained non-weight-bearing for 12 weeks or until radiographic union. Three patients were lost to follow-up, and 14 patients had less than 11 months of follow-up. Hence, 63 patients (64 fractures) with a mean follow-up of 30.3 months were evaluated in the series.

Complications included deep infection, nonunion, malunion, osteonecrosis, and posttraumatic arthritis. One deep infection occurred that resolved with debridement, irrigation, and intravenous antibiotics. Two developed malunions, and 2 developed nonunions. Thirty-five (54%) developed posttraumatic arthritis of one or more joints, and 16 (25%) developed osteonecrosis. Of the patients with osteonecrosis, the talar dome revascularized in 7 patients and collapsed in 9 patients. The mean time to radiographic signs of osteonecrosis (increased density of the talar dome) was 6.9 months.

The investigators hypothesized that the amount of initial displacement rather than timing of definitive fixation affected osteonecrosis rates. Osteonecrosis never occurred in Hawkins type I or Hawkins type IIA fractures, but occurred in 25% of Hawkins type IIB, 41% in Hawkins type III, and 33% in Hawkins type IV. The overall rate of osteonecrosis was 25% (16/23). The time of injury to emergent reduction within 6 hours, 8 hours, 12 hours, or 18 hours did not correlate with osteonecrosis, and the time to definitive fixation did not correlate with higher AVN rates. In fact, the patients that developed osteonecrosis underwent ORIF much earlier than those without osteonecrosis (1.7 days vs 4.8 days; *P*<.001). Ten Hawkins type IIB and 10 Hawkins type III fractures were treated with emergent reduction combined with delayed fixation. Of these 20, only 1 developed AVN.[3]

The aforementioned clinical research suggests the timing to definitive surgical fixation does not affect rates of osteonecrosis, union, or need for secondary reconstructive procedures. This research indicates complication rates correlate with fracture displacement, open injuries, and amount of comminution, all of which increase with the amount of traumatic force. However, these studies are retrospective with small patient populations, limiting the necessary statistical power to reject the correlation between surgical timing and complication rates (ie, type II error). Despite these limitations, these studies do demonstrate that acceptable outcomes are achievable with delayed fixation, suggesting displaced talar neck and body fractures are not inherent surgical emergencies. (**Fig. 7**)

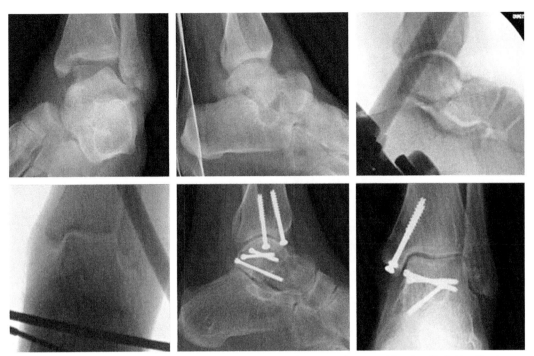

Fig. 7. Displaced talar body fracture treated with emergent reduction and external fixation. Definitive fixation was delayed for 17 days. At 18 months from injury, no signs of osteonecrosis exist on radiographs.

TALAR BODY FRACTURE VARIANTS (PROCESS AND OSTEOCHONDRAL FRACTURES)

Lateral Process Fractures

Fractures of the lateral process are frequently overlooked as simple ankle sprains, but these fractures can cause debilitating pain. Fortunately, the incidence is relatively rare in ankle injuries.[24] The lateral process involves both the tibiotalar joint at the fibular articulation and the subtalar joint at the posterior facet. The talocalcaneal, anterior talofibular, and posterior talofibular ligaments originate from the tip of the lateral process, providing stability to the ankle joint.[25,26] Historically, the mechanism of injury involves the foot dorsiflexed and inverted with an axial load,[22,27] but more recent cadaveric studies have reproduced lateral process fractures in dorsiflexed and everted or external rotated feet.[28,29] Occurring more frequently in snowboarders, these injuries represent 15% of all ankle injuries and 34% of ankle fractures in snowboarders.[30]

Patients present with symptoms mirroring an inversion ankle sprain with lateral ankle pain and swelling. Clinicians must maintain a high index of suspicion, especially in high-risk populations (ie, snowboarders) that exhibit tenderness to palpation just distal to the lateral malleolus. Radiographically, fractures are best visualized with an ankle mortise view, but advanced imaging (ie, CT scan or MRI) improves diagnostic accuracy and fracture characteristics.

Reported outcomes are limited to case reports and case series. Small, nondisplaced fractures can be treated with partial weight-bearing and immobilization for 6 weeks. For large, displaced fractures, ORIF is recommended (Fig. 8), but for small, displaced, or highly comminuted fractures, simple excision is recommended. Fractures are approached through a sinus tarsi incision with care to preserve soft tissue attachments, and fixation typically involves mini-fragment or headless implants. Initially unrecognized fractures with delayed treatment generally have poorer results.[31–33]

Posterior Process Fractures

Fractures of the posterior process involve posterior lateral and posterior medial tubercle fractures. The posterolateral tubercle is the larger of the 2 tubercles. The proximal surface of posterolateral tubercle is nonarticular and provides insertion for the posterior talofibular ligament and fibulotalocalcaneal ligament. The medial tubercle is of variable size and provides attachment for components of the deltoid ligament, medial talocalcaneal ligament, and the flexor hallicus longus tunnel. The inferior surface of the posterior process articulates with the posterior facet of the calcaneus.[1]

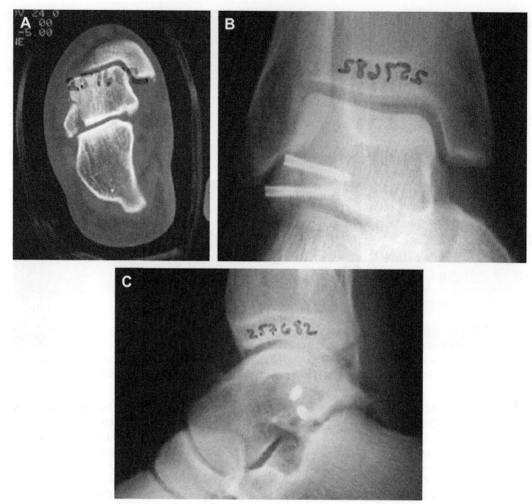

Fig. 8. (A) Displaced lateral process fracture (B, C). Lateral process fracture ORIF with headless screws. (*From* Ishikawa SN. Fractures and dislocations of the foot. In: Canale ST, Beaty JH, editors. Campbell's operative orthopaedics. 12th edition. Philadelphia: Elsevier; 2013; with permission.)

Posterolateral tubercle fractures occur with forced plantar flexion, causing direct tibial impaction,[34] or with excessive dorsiflexion, resulting in the posterior talofibular ligament avulsing the lateral tubercle.[11,35] Posteromedial tubercle avulsions transpire after forceful ankle dorsiflexion in a pronated foot.[36] Direct trauma has also been reported to cause posteromedial tubercle fractures.[37]

Radiographs typically illustrate the posterolateral tubercle well, but differentiating an acute fracture from os trigonum impingement can be difficult. With posterolateral fractures, patients present with a history of an acute ankle injury combined with significant posterior ankle pain. Alternatively, posterior impingement presents with insidious-onset, posterior ankle pain worsened with plantarflexion activities. Advanced

imaging (ie, CT scan or MRI) better characterizes the acuity, size, and displacement of posterior process fractures. Large, displaced fractures that involve a significant portion of the subtalar joint should undergo ORIF through a posterolateral approach. These fractures more truly involve the talar body proper. Otherwise, most posterolateral process fractures are typically treated conservatively with non-weight-bearing and immobilization. If conservative treatment fails, then fragment excision has shown favorable results.[38,39]

Posteromedial tubercle fractures are more difficult to visualize with radiographs, making a meticulous history and physical examination vital for accurate diagnosis (Fig. 9). After an acute injury, patients present with tenderness to palpation over the posteromedial ankle behind the

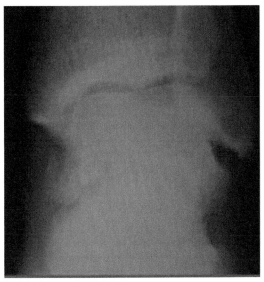
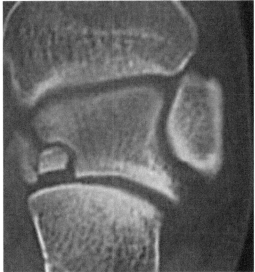

Fig. 9. Radiographic and CT imaging of posteromedial process fracture. (*From* Early JS. Talus fracture management. Foot Ankle Clin N Am 2008;13(4):652; with permission.)

medial malleolus. Nondisplaced fractures can be treated with limited weight-bearing and immobilization, but displaced fractures treated conservatively result in poor outcomes.[36,40,41] With its proximity to the tibial nerve, displaced fractures have been reported to cause tarsal tunnel symptoms.[42] Furthermore, displacement can block the movement of the subtalar joint, resulting in posttraumatic arthritis and subsequent arthrodesis. Hence, it is recommended that displaced fractures are treated with ORIF or excision.

LATERAL INVERTED OSTEOCHONDRAL FRACTURE OF THE TALUS LESIONS

Another type of body fracture often occurs in gymnasts and other jumping athletes, in which shear forces acting on the talar dome create an

acute osteochondral fracture. These lesions are often inverted, in which they are appropriately termed LIFT lesions (lateral inverted osteochondral fracture of the talus) (Fig. 10). These fractures represent an intra-articular loose body that should be treated surgically through an arthroscopic or open approach. Depending on the size of the bony fragment and the condition of the cartilage, these fractures are excised or reduced and stabilized with bioabsorbable fixation.[22,43]

TALAR EXTRUSION

Any assortment of peritalar dislocations occurs with fractures, but complete talar dislocations without fracture are extremely rare injuries. These injuries result from high-energy trauma with an

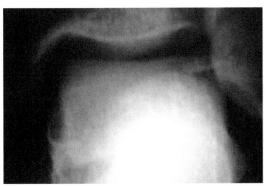
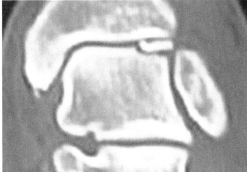

Fig. 10. Radiographic and CT imaging of LIFT lesion. (*From* Early JS. Talus fracture management. Foot Ankle Clin N Am 2008;13(4):644; with permission.)

open or intact skin envelope. Complete dislocations through an open skin wound are termed talar extrusions. Talar extrusions present a unique challenge for treating surgeons. Essentially, surgeons have the choice of reimplantation or talectomy with arthrodesis. Through case reports and small series, multiple investigators have reported favorable outcomes with talar reimplantation.[9,44–47] On the contrary, other investigators have reported poor outcomes secondary to pain, infection, and osteonecrosis, recommending primary talectomy and arthrodesis.[45,48,49] If the gross contamination can be removed, then it is generally recommended to attempt reimplantation. Before reimplantation, the talus should be treated with a 5-minute chemical soak (ie, 10% povidone-iodine or 4% Chlorhexidine) followed by a saline wash.[11,50]

SUMMARY

Fraught with disastrous complications, talar fractures continue to represent a challenging injury for orthopedic surgeons. Displaced fractures typically necessitate anatomic reduction and internal fixation to restore joint mechanics, facilitate fracture union, and allow early range of motion. Any joint dislocation should undergo emergent reduction (closed or open), but timing of definitive fixation is controversial. Recent literature demonstrates favorable outcomes with delayed fixation, suggesting that displaced talar neck and body fractures are not inherent surgical emergencies. Regardless of surgical timing, talar fractures have high complication rates, and surgeons should appropriately counsel patients about the potential sequelae from talar injuries.

REFERENCES

1. Kelikian AS, editor. Sarrafian's anatomy of the foot and ankle: descriptive, topographical, functional. 3rd edition. Philadelphia: Wolters Kluwer Health/Lippincott Williams & Wilkins; 2011. p. 48–61.
2. Farrow LD, Kimble BJ, Donley BG, et al. Unusual presentation of a talar neck fracture in an intercollegiate varsity football player. Am J Sports Med 2009;37:402–5.
3. Vallier HA, Reichard SG, Boyd AJ, et al. A new look at the Hawkins classification for talar neck fractures: which features of injury and treatment are predictive of osteonecrosis? J Bone Joint Surg Am 2014;96:192–7.
4. Hawkins LG. Fractures of the neck of the talus. J Bone Joint Surg Am 1970;52:991–1002.
5. Wildenauer E. Proceedings: Discussion on the blood supply of the talus. Z Orthop Ihre Grenzgeb 1975;113(4):730.
6. Haliburton RA, Sullivan CR, Kelly PJ, et al. The extra-osseous and intra-osseous blood supply of the talus. J Bone Joint Surg Am 1958;40-A:1115–20.
7. Gelberman RH, Mortensen WW. The arterial anatomy of the talus. Foot Ankle 1983;4:64–72.
8. Marsh JL, Slongo TF, Agel J, et al. Fracture and dislocation classification compendium—2007: Orthopaedic Trauma Association classification, database and outcomes committee. J Orthop Trauma 2007;21:S1–133.
9. Coltart WD. Aviator's astragalus. J Bone Joint Surg Br 1952;34-B:545–66.
10. Pennal GF. Fractures of the talus. Clin Orthop Relat Res 1963;30:53–63.
11. Banerjee R, Nickisch F. Fractures and fracture-dislocations of the talus. In: Coughlin MJ, Saltzman CL, Anderson RB, editors. Mann's surgery of the foot and ankle. 9th edition. Philadelphia: Elsevier; 2014. p. 2101–53.
12. Dunn AR, Jacobs B, Campbell RD Jr. Fractures of the talus. J Trauma 1966;6:443–68.
13. Kenwright J, Taylor RG. Major injuries of the talus. J Bone Joint Surg Br 1970;52:36–48.
14. Canale ST, Kelly FB Jr. Fractures of the neck of the talus. Long-term evaluation of seventy-one cases. J Bone Joint Surg Am 1978;60:143–56.
15. Penny JN, Davis LA. Fractures and fracture-dislocations of the neck of the talus. J Trauma 1980;20:1029–37.
16. Sanders DW, Busam M, Hattwick E, et al. Functional outcomes following displaced talar neck fractures. J Orthop Trauma 2004;18:265–70.
17. Vallier HA, Nork SE, Barei DP, et al. Talar neck fractures: results and outcomes. J Bone Joint Surg Am 2004;86-A:1616–24.
18. Lindvall E, Haidukewych G, DiPasquale T, et al. Open reduction and stable fixation of isolated, displaced talar neck and body fractures. J Bone Joint Surg Am 2004;86-A:2229–34.
19. Fleuriau Chateau PB, Brokaw DS, Jelen BA, et al. Plate fixation of talar neck fractures: preliminary review of a new technique in twenty-three patients. J Orthop Trauma 2002;16:213–9.
20. Swanson TV, Bray TJ, Holmes GB Jr. Fractures of the talar neck. A mechanical study of fixation. J Bone Joint Surg Am 1992;74:544–51.
21. Inokuchi S, Ogawa K, Usami N. Classification of fractures of the talus: clear differentiation between neck and body fractures. Foot Ankle Int 1996;17:748–50.
22. Early JS. Talus fracture management. Foot Ankle Clin 2008;13:635–57.
23. Vallier HA, Nork SE, Benirschke SK, et al. Surgical treatment of talar body fractures. J Bone Joint Surg Am 2003;85-A:1716–24.
24. Mukherjee SK, Young AB. Dome fracture of the talus. A report of ten cases. J Bone Joint Surg Br 1973;55:319–26.

25. Langer P, Nickisch F, Spenciner D, et al. In vitro evaluation of the effect lateral process talar excision on ankle and subtalar joint stability. Foot Ankle Int 2007;28:78–83.

26. Digiovanni CW, Langer PR, Nickisch F, et al. Proximity of the lateral talar process to the lateral stabilizing ligaments of the ankle and subtalar joint. Foot Ankle Int 2007;28:175–80.

27. Hawkins LG. Fracture of the Lateral Process of the Talus. J Bone Joint Surg Am 1965;47:1170–5.

28. Funk JR, Srinivasan SC, Crandall JR. Snowboarder's talus fractures experimentally produced by eversion and dorsiflexion. Am J Sports Med 2003;31: 921–8.

29. Boon AJ, Smith J, Zobitz ME, et al. Snowboarder's talus fracture. Mechanism of injury. Am J Sports Med 2001;29:333–8.

30. Kirkpatrick DP, Hunter RE, Janes PC, et al. The snowboarder's foot and ankle. Am J Sports Med 1998;26:271–7.

31. Von Knoch F, Reckord U, von Knoch M, et al. Fracture of the lateral process of the talus in snowboarders. J Bone Joint Surg Br 2007;89:772–7.

32. Perera A, Baker JF, Lui DF, et al. The management and outcome of lateral process fracture of the talus. Foot Ankle Surg 2010;16:15–20.

33. Valderrabano V, Perren T, Ryf C, et al. Snowboarder's talus fracture: treatment outcome of 20 cases after 3.5 years. Am J Sports Med 2005;33:871–80.

34. Hamilton WG. Stenosing tenosynovitis of the flexor hallucis longus tendon and posterior impingement upon the os trigonum in ballet dancers. Foot Ankle 1982;3:74–80.

35. Kleiger B. Injuries of the talus and its joints. Clin Orthop Relat Res 1976;(121):243–62.

36. Cedell CA. Rupture of the posterior talotibial ligament with the avulsion of a bone fragment from the talus. Acta Orthop Scand 1974;45:454–61.

37. Wolf RS, Heckman JD. Case report: fracture of the posterior medial tubercle of the talus secondary to direct trauma. Foot Ankle Int 1998;19:255–8.

38. Paulos LE, Johnson CL, Noyes FR. Posterior compartment fractures of the ankle. A commonly missed athletic injury. Am J Sports Med 1983;11: 439–43.

39. Hedrick MR, Mcbryde AM. Posterior ankle impingement. Foot Ankle Int 1994;15:2–8.

40. Ebraheim NA, Padanilam TG, Wong FY. Posteromedial process fractures of the talus. Foot Ankle Int 1995;16:734–9.

41. Kim DH, Berkowitz MJ, Pressman DN. Avulsion fractures of the medial tubercle of the posterior process of the talus. Foot Ankle Int 2003;24: 172–5.

42. Stefko RM, Lauerman WC, Heckman JD. Tarsal tunnel syndrome caused by an unrecognized fracture of the posterior process of the talus (Cedell fracture). A case report. J Bone Joint Surg Am 1994; 76:116–8.

43. Dunlap BJ, Ferkel RD, Applegate GR. The "LIFT" lesion: lateral inverted osteochondral fracture of the talus. Arthroscopy 2013;29:1826–33.

44. Ritsema GH. Total talar dislocation. J Trauma 1988; 28:692–4.

45. Hiraizumi Y, Hara T, Takahashi M, et al. Open total dislocation of the talus with extrusion (missing talus): report of two cases. Foot Ankle 1992;13: 473–7.

46. Marsh JL, Saltzman CL, Iverson M, et al. Major open injuries of the talus. J Orthop Trauma 1995;9:371–6.

47. Smith CS, Nork SE, Sangeorzan BJ. The extruded talus: results of reimplantation. J Bone Joint Surg Am 2006;88:2418–24.

48. Detenbeck LC, Kelly PJ. Total dislocation of the talus. J Bone Joint Surg Am 1969;51:283–8.

49. Jaffe KA, Conlan TK, Sardis L, et al. Traumatic talectomy without fracture: four case reports and review of the literature. Foot Ankle Int 1995;16:583–7.

50. Bruce B, Sheibani-Rad S, Appleyard D, et al. Are dropped osteoarticular bone fragments safely reimplantable in vivo? J Bone Joint Surg Am 2011;93:430–8.

Index

Note: Page numbers of article titles are in **boldface** type.

Orthop Clin N Am 47 (2016) 639–643
http://dx.doi.org/10.1016/S0030-5898(16)30029-3
0030-5898/16/$ – see front matter

Moving?

Make sure your subscription moves with you!

To notify us of your new address, find your **Clinics Account Number** (located on your mailing label above your name), and contact customer service at:

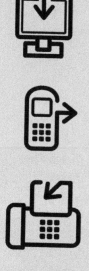

Email: journalscustomerservice-usa@elsevier.com

800-654-2452 (subscribers in the U.S. & Canada)
314-447-8871 (subscribers outside of the U.S. & Canada)

Fax number: 314-447-8029

Elsevier Health Sciences Division
Subscription Customer Service
3251 Riverport Lane
Maryland Heights, MO 63043

*To ensure uninterrupted delivery of your subscription, please notify us at least 4 weeks in advance of move.

ELSEVIER